Champions Needed

Unlocking the Potential of Family Advocacy in Assisted Living and Memory Care

Artell Smith

with

Carol J. Purdy Miller

Foreword by Lois C. Smith, Ph.D.

i

CHAMPIONS NEEDED

Unlocking the Potential of Family Advocacy
in Assisted Living and Memory Care

Table of Contents

Legal Disclaimer

We're not lawyers; this work does not contain legal advice. Every situation is unique, varying with the organizations, people, facts, and circumstances. Contact a licensed lawyer for legal counsel if deemed necessary. Stories, examples, and suggestions contained in *Champions Needed* arise from the authors' experiences, observations, and research. To ensure anonymity, we have changed story details. The examples we use are intended only to illustrate the content expressed. Any resemblance to actual organizations or anyone living or deceased is coincidental. Permission has been obtained to recount a story as a whole or in part if needed. We're not critics; we're advocates.

With Thanks

With Thanks and In Memoriam to Artell's mother Lois C. Smith (1935-2024) who made her transition shortly after writing her Forward to Champions Needed. "God gave me an angel and her name was mom." Mom-because of your life, love, generosity, success, inspiration and example, I'm who I am today. I love you, will remember you fondly, and eternally miss you.

To Artell's wife, Susan Burns Smith, who greets every day as a new adventure.

To Carol's mother, Mary Lois Purdy, who is a constant inspiration, source of joy and a companion on new ventures.

And to Steve King, who planted the seed for this book in Artell's mind on a sunny October day in Madison, WI

About the Authors

Artell Smith

Artell has spent nearly 40 years as a Human Resources professional in several large and complex organizations. He's retired twice thus far and is working on his third—still several years away. Artell is an adjunct instructor at the Center for Professional and Executive Development, Wisconsin School of Business at the University of Wisconsin–Madison. Over the past decade, he has taught hundreds of managers, leaders, and executives critical skills to become more effective. Artell's interest in the care of seniors in assisted living and memory care communities arose from the experiences of two of his loved ones, his wife and mother. Respectively, Artell's wife, Susan, lives in a memory care community, and his mother, Lois, lives in an assisted living community. Along with other family members, Artell plays the health and well-being advocate role for his wife and mother. He's the author of *No Time to Waste—Microbehaviors: Leveraging the Little Things to Become a Better Leader* (April 2023) and *Engage.Coach.Develop: Building Strong Relationships That Drive Individual and Team Performance* (October 2023). Artell is also the author of two works of fiction, one written with his son Troy. He holds a B.A. and a Master of Public Administration from Brigham Young University. Artell lives in Southeast Wisconsin near the shores of Lake Michigan.

Carol J. Purdy Miller

Carol is a retired educator, health care & food services administrator, and registered dietitian. For 23 years, she served as an officer in the United States military with assignments at Brooke Army Medical Center, Fort Campbell, Walter Reed Army Medical Center, Fitzsimmons Army Medical Center, and The Pentagon, among others. After retiring from the military, Carol worked in food service administration, retiring again from Colorado's sixth-largest K-12 school district and various management roles in private business. She served in numerous professional organizations and mentored

Graduate Dietetic Students at Colorado State University and the University of Northern Colorado. In addition, Carol taught nutrition at Front Range Community College. Her interest in seniors' care stems from the care experiences of her father and mother. With other family members, Carol plays the role of health and well-being advocate for her mother, Lois, who lives in an independent-plus apartment. Carol holds a B.S. from the University of Illinois (Urbana), a Master of Systems Management from USC, and a Master of Health Care Administration from Baylor University. Carol and her husband, C.W., live in the picturesque mountain foothills near Bellvue, Colorado.

Foreword

Artell and Carol asked me to write the Foreword to *Champions Needed: Unlocking the Potential of Family Advocacy in Assisted Living and Memory Care* since I am a long-term care community resident and have experience with health care and well-being champions. Over the past five years, I have lived in several assisted living communities in two States. Most of the time, my daily journey goes smoothly. But there are bumps in the road—more and more of them, it seems--that require the help of community staff to be accomplished. This is not ideal for me; it offends my sense of who I am and dramatically diminishes the independence I once enjoyed.

I was educated as a scientist and hold a Ph.D. in Chemistry from Rutgers University. I also have a master's degree from the University of Illinois (Urbana) and a bachelor's degree from Douglass College. My parents, Frank and Clara Crisbacher, raised me to be self-sufficient, and so I have been for nearly all my long life.

My husband, Franklin Artell Smith, was also a scientist with a Ph.D. in Chemistry from a German university. We met in a large pharmaceutical company's laboratory and were blessed with four children: Paul (aka Artell), Philip, Jennifer, and Stephen. Unlike my husband, I did not want to make my career in pharmaceuticals and felt my calling to be in academia.

Leaving the commercial business setting, I was hired as an Assistant Professor of Chemistry in 1964 at Russell Sage College in Troy, New York. Over my 16 years at Sage, I was promoted to Professor of Chemistry and Department Chair. My last position at the college was as Academic Dean. To advance my career further, I left Sage and moved to Ithaca College as Provost. Later, I served as chief academic officer at East Stroudsburg State University and Texas Woman's University.

Upon retirement in 2004, I moved to Spencer, New York, living in a small home on eight wooded acres. I was able to take care of myself until a diagnosis of Parkinson's Disease, with the accompanying physical challenges, required a move into an assisted living community. That happened in December 2018, and I haven't laid eyes on my house since I was taken to the hospital on a cold Sunday morning.

The move to assisted living was an abrupt and anxiety-provoking event despite the best efforts of my children, particularly my son Philip. While I was prepared financially, it was physically and mentally demanding. I am not sure I can claim to be over those challenging events, but I can now look beyond them.

Let me address the most critical issue I want to comment on in this Foreword. Namely, all assisted living community residents should have an advocate to champion their healthcare needs and help deal with complex organizational structures.

My failing physical health, including decreased mobility combined with hearing and vision loss, makes it impossible for me to tend to the many details of confinement to assisted living. In those first years, my advocate, Philip, was in constant dialog with the community's administrative and caregiving staff. He worked tirelessly to balance suggestions for improvements versus simply registering complaints.

The basic skills healthcare and well-being advocates need are compassion, empathy, active listening, negotiations, problem-solving, and conflict resolution. All assisted living residents, me included, crave the ability to count on continuous, consistent care without reminding community staff of what needs to be done. These are essential requirements for a buyer and consumer of assisted living services. I have yet to enjoy the continuity and consistency of care I expect in all cases. In my experience, many small and significant care points must be reviewed multiple times before they're correctly rendered. Again, an advocate is required.

However, I am not here to point fingers or assign blame. I cannot make a window into the souls of administrators and caregivers to ascertain their full intentions. I can only experience and then judge the behaviors around me. The world is an uncertain place, as we all know. Not being able to address my desires and needs independently makes the uncertainty occasionally frustrating. Having someone by my side, advocating for my health care needs, lessens the uncertainty, allowing for more pleasant moments to accumulate.

A true partnership with my healthcare and well-being advocate is needed based on mutual trust and respect. In my case, my children do this for me. However, a family advocate(s) is not always available. It might need to be a friend. Whatever the case, advocates need skills and patience to perform their duties well.

This book, authored by Artell and Carol, offers practical tips for becoming an effective advocate for your loved one in assisted living or memory care. As an educator, I know we can learn new things if we're willing. If you are not the advocate you want to be or need to be, spending time with this book is an excellent way to sharpen your skills.

Lois C. Smith, Ph.D.
Former Professor of Chemistry and Academic Administrator
Current Assisted Living Community Resident
Kenosha, Wisconsin

Prologue

The specter of older adults being placed into a nursing home to spend the rest of their days unhappily is part of our cultural story. *The Simpsons* have used the Grandpa character for over thirty years to make this point. Gabe Simpson's send-ups of life *down to the home* have elicited many laughs from us. Perhaps from you, too.

As we've grown older, we don't laugh as much at Grandpa's commentary about *the home.* The possibility of being *sent* to a long-term care community by well-intentioned but possibly tone-deaf relatives is more concerning to us nowadays. We recall visiting older relatives in nursing homes when we were young. We had the impression from our parents, uncles, aunts, and others that these places were not desirable but necessary. To us, they were dark, brooding, and smelled funny.

As a society, we've become somewhat more empathetic and now boast several options for seniors to fit their circumstances as they age. The various possibilities can be fitted along the now-fashionable *continuum of care* spectrum. Independent living is followed by independent-plus assisted living, memory care, and skilled nursing care. Not everyone starts with independent living, nor ends with skilled nursing care. The guiding principle is that the best living arrangement for a senior loved one is based on the needs of the individual.[1]

But how should the decision be made? What criteria should be used? Who makes the final determination? How much say should family members have versus the loved ones who are directly impacted? And what of the comfortable, familiar house or apartment that is left behind? And what of the belongings contained within it? There are a myriad of issues and questions, both large and small.

---

[1] For an extended discussion of various possible living arrangements, see Chapter 2, Fundamentals of the Long-Term Care Industry.

For *Champions Needed*, we assume the decision to move a loved one to a long-term care community has already been made. That your loved one is, or will be soon, living in independent living, independent-plus assisted living, memory care, or skilled nursing care. But you may be in the exploration stage, and a firm decision has yet to be made. If that's the case, we think you'll still find this book useful since the skills of a healthcare advocate or champion are much the same, regardless of the setting.

We can point you to the wisdom of many experts who have thought deeply about the most important considerations as you weigh options for your loved ones. We have cited available resources and provided some of our thoughts in the End Notes and Tools section under *Choosing a Long-Term Care Community*.

Chapter 1—Senior Loved Ones Deserve Our Best

Why we're writing this book

We're writing this book because we believe our senior loved ones living in long-term care communities—particularly independent-plus, assisted living, and memory care—need the best from those around them at a time when their ability to advocate and care for themselves has diminished. It's not because they don't want to continue to be their own spokespersons and live independently; it's just increasingly difficult to do so.

We focused on independent-plus, assisted living, and memory care communities partly because we're most comfortable in this space and generally possess more expertise. Skilled nursing care communities have similar missions, and advocate/champion skills are essentially the same. Still, those specialized communities require a different focus and often a more watchful approach from the advocate.

In *Champions Needed*, we use the terms *advocate* and *champion* interchangeably to highlight their importance in supporting seniors. Champions are instrumental in ensuring seniors receive the necessary protections, care, and resources, regardless of their living situation. Advocacy isn't limited to professionals; family, friends, and even trusted colleagues can take on this role.

The positive impact of advocacy is evident, especially for seniors who cannot advocate for themselves. Effective advocacy involves constant communication with a loved one's care team, sharing updates about their changing needs or preferences, and ensuring their personal beliefs are respected.

When seniors partner with a champion, they benefit from a more engaged and individualized approach to care and decision-making. Although it's beneficial to have an advocate, empowering loved ones to speak up for themselves for as long as possible is essential. Advocates can encourage loved ones to suggest the best person to approach if they don't wish to speak on their behalf.

In memory care, as cognitive and physical decline progresses, an advocate becomes the loved one's voice, articulating their wishes when they cannot. A champion who knows their loved one well can provide essential insights to tailor the care plans to the individual's unique needs and history. This personalized approach ensures that even as memory fades, the dignity and individuality of the person are being honored.

We aren't here as critics of long-term care communities

Before we continue, a caveat: Much has been written about long-term care communities' challenges, especially since the first Boomer turned 65 in 2010. However, our purpose in writing *Champions Needed* is not to point fingers at the industry or specific communities. Instead, we wish to encourage individuals and families to prepare themselves more thoroughly to become effective champions for loved ones who can no longer manage independently. Whatever the reality is within the operating confines of a long-term care community, skilled advocates can make a difference.

We applaud the efforts of government, private, and non-profit organizations to ensure long-term care communities are meeting quality standards. They play a crucial role in ascertaining whether they're living up to the trust placed in them by residents, their families, and the public in general. We leave it to these watchdog organizations to point out weaknesses, failure points, and areas of immediate improvement.

Definition of advocate/champion

An advocate/champion relinquishes a portion of their freedom to be a vocal proponent of someone else's needs. We're not speaking of a *caregiver* since that's one step beyond an advocate, though some people answer the call to be both. Instead, we're talking about a person, whether a family member or friend, who takes on the privilege of continuously championing the cause of a loved one through whatever stages of care they may need.

The job of a champion is difficult. To succeed, the person must become skilled in many esoteric human interaction arts, including communication, emotional intelligence, conflict management, problem-solving, and many other active skills. If a designated advocate still needs to gain the necessary life skills to play the role, they must become agile learners.

We're both advocates and can confirm without hesitation it's among the most challenging and satisfying roles we've ever played, personal or professional. The reason? A loved one's quality of life depends on us—not in a symbolic way but in a literal way. Poor advocacy for a loved one in a long-term care community has immediate and sometimes life-threatening consequences.

Deep emotion and feelings are part and parcel of being a champion. How many of us could stand indifferently if we saw a loved one struggling in an environment that could be improved if we only acted? We know we couldn't. And you probably couldn't either.

An advocate or champion is a *dedicated sponsor* of a loved one in a long-term care community. We can also use the labels cheerleader, promoter, or supporter as applicable synonyms. An advocate/champion vigorously assists and has an active, ongoing role in backing the loved one's health and well-being. There is no adequate substitute for a vocal advocate; even though a champion is a *single voice* in a noisy environment, your loved one benefits from your efforts.

Remember, moving a loved one into a community generally results from a valid reason, which means change for everyone. This could cause personal guilt if you're involved in the decision to move your loved one. While it's beyond the scope of this book, the loved one must be shielded from your issues. A loved one may also feel like they're being dumped into a long-term care community. Champions must try to assuage this belief and strike a positive note in all possible ways.

Success through a series of positive actions

Championing connotes deliberate *action*. Advocates are constantly in motion, observing, questioning, recommending, and persisting—another way to describe advocating and championing as a verb is to visualize *standing up* for someone else. We like the verticality of standing up since it implies forward progress, which is the desired outcome of proper advocacy. Now that you've read a little about the context of this book, here's what we hope you'll gain from reading it.

1) **A clear understanding of the role and responsibilities of an advocate**—the accountabilities you should expect to shoulder and the typical tasks that must be accomplished on behalf of your loved one.
2) **A general grasp of the skills, knowledge, and abilities required of a champion**—the behaviors to improve the life of your loved one. And the importance of being an agile learner.
3) **An appreciation of how to move forward quickly through various common scenarios**—the strategies that will meet your objectives while building relationships with those who provide caregiving services for your loved one.

You may feel a bit overwhelmed as you embark on fulfilling the duties of a champion. Recall you already have many skills required through your personal life experiences (as a parent, brother, sister, uncle, or aunt, for example) that will transfer to becoming an effective advocate, perhaps with only a few adjustments. Once modified, skills application in new ways will become easy with experience and time.

Consider: if you've been advocating for a loved one who lived with you or nearby, the skills employed may continue to be necessary. For example, you may no longer need to shop for or cook your loved one's meals, but you may still need to review community menus to ensure proper nutrition. Or, if you've assured your loved one is appropriately taking medications or prescriptions, changes were implemented correctly and continue.

True stories: some facts intentionally changed

We have stories to tell from our own experiences and the experiences of people in our networks, some of whom are residents of long-term care communities and some of whom are champions for those who are. In all cases, we'll protect the anonymity of people and communities in our stories.

In that spirit, we have our first story to share. One that starts us off on a positive note and showcases the vital role a champion can play.

We know loved ones who felt they were being roughly treated by a caregiver during transfers from bed to wheelchair to bathroom and then back again. The loved one voiced their concerns to the caregiver but was rebuffed. The loved one was reluctant to escalate further for fear of being labeled a troublemaker, but they did tell their advocate.

However, the champion saw the risk of poorly executed transfers and decided to step in personally. The champion contacted the community's human resources representative, described the situation, and requested an investigation. The HR representative interviewed the loved one, with the champion present, and the employee was ultimately disciplined.

Despite the loved one's worries, an advocate doesn't have the option to do nothing. In our view, the absence of action creates a void in which chaos thrives.

Stephen Hawking said:

Chaos, when left alone, tends to multiply.[2]

---

2 "Stephen Hawking Quote: 'Chaos, When Left Alone, Tends to Multiply.,'"
n.d. https://quotefancy.com/quote/910026/Stephen-Hawking-Chaos-when-left-alone-tends-to-multiply.

NOTES

Chapter 2—Fundamentals of the Long-Term Care Industry

Becoming an effective champion for your loved one in need of long-term care requires a fundamental understanding of the available options for seniors. This chapter will briefly cover the critical differences between the types of senior communities and the residents they serve.

At the outset of this analysis, we want to state that the word *facility* has fallen out of favor over time. Instead, we use the word *community* since it more aptly characterizes the intent, if not always the reality, of where your loved one lives. This is tricky terminology despite the apparent nature of the difference between a facility and a community.

In our minds, the facility language identifies a *place,* while the community language identifies a *state of mind.* Your loved one lives in a facility with an address but is hopeful that the experience transcends the uniformly beige walls, white miniblinds, and taupe carpeting. The essence of the advocacy role is to ensure every new day includes friendship and camaraderie with fellow community residents and an enthusiasm—albeit subdued—for life in general.

For-profit versus non-profit communities

Before we present the definitions of the various types of communities, it's essential to understand the difference between a community run on a for-profit basis versus a community run on a non-profit basis.

In the U.S., over 80% of long-term care communities are run for profit.[3] This means the *bottom line* matters greatly, where expenses are managed carefully to achieve a surplus or a profit. The services

---

[3] Samuels, Claire. "Assisted Living Statistics: Population & Facilities in 2023." A Place for Mom, December 5, 2023. https://www.aplaceformom.com/senior-living-data/articles/assisted-living-statistics.

provided by for-profit versus non-profit entities are essentially the same. While the emphasis is always on delivering high-quality services, there is also a deep focus on managing costs in a for-profit establishment.

In theory, a community run on a non-profit basis takes the annual surplus and reinvests it back into the community. The evidence of this happening should be higher staff-to-resident ratios and higher quality of service. However, there needs to be more evidence that this is the case since high-quality and low-quality communities can be found in relatively equal proportions of for-profit and non-profit spaces.

Some non-profit communities may appeal to you and your loved one simply because they're smaller and more personalized. There also may be a difference in cost, which, of course, is highly dependent on the total number of well-trained staff. The decision to place a loved one in a for-profit or non-profit community will come down to the specifics of daily life and financial means. Again, the nature and quality of care are the same.

Continuum of care communities

First, we want to discuss the continuum of care community concept. This idea or philosophy is also referred to as *aging in place*. It's most definitely not a new idea. But these types of communities are becoming much more common. The early period of investigating how seniors could age in place occurred between 1979 and 1985. In the mid-1980s, servicing models existed on the U.S.'s East and West coasts, primarily Oregon and Virginia, among other forward-thinking States. For more in-depth information, we recommend looking up the seminal 2007 work of Keren Brown Wilson and her article titled *Historical Evolution of Assisted Living in the United States, 1979 to the Present.*[4]

What arose from this and the following periods of evolution for assisted living was the idea that a range of care options was needed

---

[4] Wilson, Keren Brown. "Historical Evolution of Assisted Living in the United States, 1979 to the Present." *The Gerontologist* 47, no. suppl_1 (December 1, 2007): 8–22. https://doi.org/10.1093/geront/47.supplement_1.8.

in *one community.* Baby Boomers led the way, first for their parents and then for themselves.

There is substantial value in an aging-in-place community, mainly when all care levels are on the same campus and staff rotates through the differing care levels. Moving a resident into an aging-in-place community will be less traumatic for everyone. Many things about and in the community are well-known; administrative and financial requirements have been completed, and the physical moving process is more straightforward.

In the U.S., many communities now advertise themselves as *ideal* places for seniors to age in place. We're still determining if the word *ideal* should be used with such abandon. We can say with certainty that all communities, whether specialized or aspiring to provide the elusive continuum of care, require continued vigilance from advocates for loved ones. What's critical here is that champions must learn how the individual community's systems work and be prepared to intervene in many ways and at all levels.

Independent living communities

A typical independent living community member is a person 55 years of age and older who is mentally and physically able to live alone without skilled health care or assistance with Activities of Daily Living (ADLs). There are two types of independent living residences. First, fit-for-purpose patio homes or apartment complexes explicitly designed for qualified seniors who are tired of maintaining their homes and yards but choose to live independently with no additional services. Second, an independent senior living apartment with individual suites for a loved one who is weary of cooking food, worried about personal safety, and seeking regular social interaction. In this second option, unfurnished senior-adapted apartments frequently include grab bars, walk-/roll-in showers, wheelchair accessibility, vehicle parking, gathering areas, dining room meals, scheduled social activities, and transportation.

An emerging approach within independent living communities is the *independent-plus* option, a service extension catering to seniors who desire added conveniences and assistance in their apartments. This hybrid model includes services such as personal laundry, bed linen changes, and housekeeping—amenities enhancing everyday living—supplemented with some ADL assistance and medication management.

To further tailor these services, healthcare staff within the community assess your loved one's needs focused on ADLs like dressing, eating, bathing, and medication management before move-in. The assessment outcome determines the level of care required, which then determines the level of care and, thus, additional monthly costs (generally tax deductible). Should your loved one's needs progress to the point where continuous oversight due to conditions such as incontinence or reduced mobility becomes necessary, it may become compulsory to transfer your loved one to a different area of the community or possibly to a new community.

Available services vary widely by community and the number of residents. Some independent living communities may even offer on-site or contracted therapeutic services such as medical care, monthly wellness checks, a podiatrist for toenail trimming, PT, OT, and speech therapies, eliminating the need for your loved one to drive. Add-on services may be billed to Medicare or supplemental health insurance, or you can expect to pay incrementally higher monthly rent.

Some independent-plus assisted living residents may prefer to obtain such assistance through third-party services. With 10,000 Baby Boomers turning 65 *every day*, you can see why so many options exist within this category. Aging Baby Boomers will further influence the future construction of independent living communities.

Assisted living communities

An assisted living community is a residential option for a loved one who needs substantial help with daily routines and mobility, including ADLs. Services offered are designed to help residents maintain as much independence and personal dignity as possible. All the services provided by independent living communities can and should be found in assisted living communities.

Medication management is generally a hallmark of assisted living arrangements and is essential for an advocate's peace of mind. Adhering to medication administration schedules is a common challenge for seniors. Assisted living provides increased structure and routine, allowing for greater enjoyment of life.

Assisted living communities are generally licensed at the state level and have regulations that focus on the well-being and safety of residents. Staff may include personal care assistants and licensed nurses, but medical care is less intensive than in memory care or skilled nursing care communities.

Memory care communities

A memory care community is a residential option for a loved one who suffers from memory impairment, like Alzheimer's or generalized dementia. While memory impairment strikes at any age, most people who require this advanced care level are 65 and older. In 2023, 10.7% of the U.S. population (1 in 9 or 6.7 million people) in the 65+ age group suffer from Alzheimer's or other forms of dementia.[5]

Cognitive impairment is usually mild initially but can grow to the point where the individual can no longer perform routine tasks without prompting, directing, or assisting. You probably have at least one older family member who fits into this demographic and already understands what's needed for ongoing care. The services provided in both independent and assisted living are frequently the same as what's provided in a memory care community. The ability to reason and act independently is what's *lost* by your loved one, therefore placing greater accountability on the shoulders of a champion.

Memory care communities often fall under similar licensing as assisted living facilities but may have additional requirements due to the specialized nature of their care. Staff typically undergo specific

---

[5] Alzheimer's Association. "2023 ALZHEIMER'S DISEASE FACTS AND FIGURES SPECIAL REPORT THE PATIENT JOURNEY IN AN ERA OF NEW TREATMENTS." *Https://Www.Alz.Org/Alzheimers-Dementia/Facts-Figures*. Alzheimer's Association, 2023. https://doi.org/10.1002/alz.13016.

training for dementia care, and the community might need to meet detailed design and security standards to create a safe environment for residents.

Skilled nursing care communities

A skilled nursing care community is a residential option for a loved one who requires round-the-clock, ongoing, skilled services delivered by licensed healthcare professionals. Nursing care communities provide long-term care for seniors and others with severe health conditions, rehabilitative care post-surgery, fractures, hospitalization, significant illness, and hospice.

Nursing care communities are designed for people who cannot manage daily activities and require more medical attention or rehabilitation than those provided in an assisted living or memory care community. Services provided to residents typically involve wound care, intravenous therapy, and monitoring of vital signs and medical equipment.

Skilled nursing communities and their facilities require a higher level of licensing due to the necessary medical services. If they accept Medicare and Medicaid patients, both federal and state laws regulate them. Strict health and safety regulations must be followed. Qualified staff often include nurse practitioners, registered nurses, licensed practical nurses, and certified nurse aides.

Long-term care industry challenges

As is the case with all areas of economic endeavor, there are several challenges the senior caregiving industry presently faces. We point out these issues purely as a way for advocates to become fully prepared for their duties. Similar headwinds can be found in any economic endeavor where money is exchanged for services. If you've recently been disappointed in service at your local restaurant, car dealership, educational institution, or credit card company, you know what we're talking about. Here are four long-term trends that will continue to beset the industry into the foreseeable future:

- **Recruitment and retention**—Since before the pandemic, almost all organizations providing health services have been chronically understaffed and unable to keep up with growing demand. This is not a unique problem but one found in nearly all industries. The U.S. has enjoyed very low unemployment for over a decade, other than a notable uptick during the pandemic, and as of December 2023, the unemployment rate stood at 3.7%.[6] Staff recruitment in assisted living, memory care, and nursing care communities suffer as much as other sectors due to the general labor shortage.

  On the flip side of the recruitment challenge is the retention challenge. This is partly due to overall low unemployment as described but is exacerbated by staff members' perceptions about wages, working conditions, shift schedules, overtime hours, treatment by management, and interactions with residents and their family members. While most of these workplace issues are not unique, there is an emotional poignance component in long-term care environments that is hard to appreciate until experienced directly by staff. Many workers are just not cut out to be in long-term care roles. But that's a matter of opinion.

What does it mean for you as an advocate?

  - Staff member turnover *will* be high.
  - Finding replacements *will* take longer than you think reasonable.
  - Repeated explanations of your loved one's situation *will* be needed.
  - Staff *will* suffer burnout, and care lapses *will* occur.

- **Senior population increase**—The number of individuals who reached the remarkable age of 100 stood at about 90,000 in 2021, double what it was 20 years earlier. Many public health initiatives in the U.S. beginning in 1900 have contributed to overall longevity, like adding chlorine to water supplies and the improved availability of prenatal care, smoking cessation, and

---

[6] For the most up-to-date information on U.S. unemployment, visit the Department of Labor, Bureau of Labor Statistics website at https://www.bls.gov.

disease elimination (polio, smallpox, TB). Healthcare treatments and technology improved the chances of living to ripe old age.

However, the most crucial reason for the dramatic increase in centenarians and all other 65 and older age groups is the total size of the post-World War II *Baby Boom.*[7] As of the 2020 census, roughly 55.5 million people were 65 or older, representing one in every six in the country. Between 2010 and 2020, this population grew by 38.6% vs. 7.4% for the U.S. as a whole.[8]

The vast Baby Boomer population is entering and progressing through senior living communities. By 2030, the population of seniors will grow to one in every five people in the U.S., and seven out of ten seniors will require long-term care services. Such dramatic changes will significantly increase demand and stress the industry for 20-30 years.

What does it mean for you as an advocate?

- There *will* be increasing competition for community openings.
- Your loved one's longevity and inevitable decline *will* burden you more.
- Senior loved ones *will* look to your expertise to become their advocate.
- Your personal health issues will multiply as you age, potentially making it difficult to be an advocate.

- **Generational group differences**—You have likely heard these terms used as shorthand descriptions of generations: Baby Boomers, Gen X, Millennials, Gen Z, and perhaps even Gen Alpha. Most researchers approach delineating one generation from another based on a date range. The span of years is usually a 15 to 20-year period.

---

[7] O'Connell-Domenech, Alejandra. "The Hill." *The Hill,* February 7, 2023. https://thehill.com/changing-america/well-being/longevity/3847532-more-people-are-living-to-be-100-heres-why/.

[8] US Census Bureau, "U.S. Older Population Grew from 2010 to 2020 at Fastest Rate since 1880 to 1890," Census.gov, May 25, 2023, https://www.census.gov/library/stories/2023/05/2020-census-united-states-older-population-grew.html.

However, experts agree there is no distinct beginning or ending to a generation grouping since the generation you *claim* may differ from the timespan during which you were born. According to Dr. Deborah, most generational mindsets arise from critical, historical events, first provoking a transitional period at the end of one generational grouping followed by a more cohesive *new* generation. [9] [10]

Long-term care communities are challenged by the natural mindset differences between caregivers and those being cared for. In one situation, a competent caregiver was 70 years younger than the resident who depended on them for help. There is no reason for the age difference to matter, provided the young caregiver did their job competently. And yet, the seven decades of age difference did make a difference in the comfort level of the senior loved one and their champion.

What does it mean for you as an advocate?

- You need to be aware of your generational biases.
- Recognize everyone is an individual with the potential to learn and grow.
- Find common ground, generational *safe places*.
- You should do more research on generational mindset differences.

- **Cost of care**—It would be tough to live in the U.S. without coming to the grim conclusion that healthcare costs are very high and rising faster than the overall inflation rate. From 2000 to 2022, the overall price of consumer goods and services increased by 80.8%. In comparison, the cost of medical care (including insurance, prescription drugs, and medical equipment) increased

---

[9] Geiger, Abigail. "The Whys and Hows of Generations Research | Pew Research Center." Pew Research Center - U.S. Politics & Policy, May 22, 2023. https://www.pewresearch.org/politics/2015/09/03/the-whys-and-hows-of-generations-research/.

[10] Cottrell, Sarah. "A Year-by-Year Guide to the Different Generations." *Parents*, January 30, 2024. https://www.parents.com/parenting/better-parenting/style/generation-names-and-years-a-cheat-sheet-for-parents/.

by 114.3%.[11] A 33.5% difference! While there was some relief in this trend for 2023, estimates of future growth suggest Americans will continue to see medical costs rise faster than other goods and services.

Long-term care costs, including assisted living, memory care, and nursing care, generally rise faster than medical costs. Our research discovered no standard way to measure long-term care cost increases. Still, there is general agreement across many government and independent research studies indicating Baby Boomers are unprepared for this type of expense.[12]

Organizations operating long-term care communities respond to supply and demand like other industries. Boomers drive demand, and the supply needs to grow faster. *A perfect storm for consumers has arrived*. In 2021, more than half of assisted living communities in the U.S. cost $54,000 annually, with prices rising steeply closer to central metropolitan areas. Locked memory care units can easily be double that amount. Providers driven by a profit motive will continue to push these annual expenses higher in the coming years.[13]

What does it mean for you as an advocate?

- You may be called upon to contribute to your loved one's expenses.
- If employed, your ability to perform your work effectively may diminish.
- Your retirement plans may be disrupted or delayed.

---

[11] Peterson-KFF Health System Tracker. "How Does Medical Inflation Compare to Inflation in the Rest of the Economy? - Peterson-KFF Health System Tracker," July 31, 2023. https://www.healthsystemtracker.org/brief/how-does-medical-inflation-compare-to-inflation-in-the-rest-of-the-economy/
[12] Rowland, Christopher. "Senior Care Is Crushingly Expensive. Boomers Aren't Ready." *Washington Post*, March 24, 2023. https://www.washingtonpost.com/business/2023/03/18/senior-care-costs-too-high/.
[13] Rau, Reed Abelson New York Times, Jordan. "Facing Financial Ruin as Costs Soar for Elder Care - KFF Health News." KFF Health News, December 4, 2023.

- You'll find it increasingly difficult to endure poor-quality service incidents.

- **Caregiver training**—The Federal government does not regulate caregiver training in assisted living or memory care communities. However, the Federal Centers for Medicare and Medicaid Services (CMS) promulgates minimum standards for skilled nursing communities. Rules and training standards for assisted living and memory care are handled state-by-state with no common reference point.[14] However, industry groups and watchdog organizations have put forward some best practice proposals for state and local governments to consider.[15]

  Note: The licensure of Registered Nurses (RNs) and Licensed Practical Nurses (LPNs) is highly regulated and rigorously policed. Our use of the word caregiver does not include RNs or LPNs. For detailed information on nursing licensure, please see the National Council of State Boards of Nursing, Inc. website—www.ncsbn.org.

  Requirements for caregiver training vary significantly at the state level and are frequently rudimentary. Community administrative leaders are concerned about the quality of care and make substantial efforts to train staff initially and over time. Nevertheless, this is challenging for communities given the other headwinds they face, like recruitment, retention, and controlling the cost of care, discussed earlier in this chapter. See the End Notes and Tools section at the back for a complete list of essential training topics.

---

[14] Schier-Akamelu, Rebecca. "What Are the State Requirements for Assisted Living Communities? An Overview," January 8, 2024. https://www.aplaceformom.com/caregiver-resources/articles/assisted-living-violations.

[15] Mollot, Richard J, JD, Sean Whang MPH, Dara Valanejad JD, and The Long-Term Care Community Coalition. *Assisted Living: Promising Policies and Practices for Improving Resident Health, Quality of Life, and Safety*. eBook. New York, United States of America: The Long-Term Care Community Coalition, 2018. https://nursinghome411.org/ltccc-report-assisted-living-promising-policies-and-practices/.

What does it mean for you as an advocate?

- Prepare mentally and emotionally for variations in caregivers' skill sets, commitment, and personalities.
- Anticipate your loved one will experience errors of omission and commission.
- Recognize caregivers may have minimal awareness of their skill gaps.
- Understand where you *draw the line* between essential and non-essential skills.

Neither friend nor foe—it's a job

One of our mothers recently commented she'd not seen a particular caregiver for over a week and wondered when they would return to the community. *Perhaps they're on vacation or sick,* she ventured. A few days after she commented, we learned the caregiver had resigned and moved on to other things. The mom was distressed since the caregiver was very good at the job, and she would miss them. She was also surprised that the caregiver had not said goodbye since their relationship was very personal, given the daily help she received.

Over our careers, we've both held positions that included managing others. Sometimes, we've been sad to see someone leave their job for a better opportunity. Such things happen. But it was emotionally challenging the first few times we'd lost an employee from the workplace, of whom we'd grown fond.

Some questions arose:

- Didn't they enjoy working with us as much as we enjoyed working with them?
- Weren't we friends at some level?
- Hadn't we spent hours and hours with them?
- Wasn't our mentorship and training valued?

Possible answers are *yes, no, and maybe,* plus many variations!

Work friends are a particular category of friendship that frequently has a definite beginning and end. The comings and goings in any organization are times for celebration and sadness. Then, everyone moves on.

The problem in long-term care is there is a third person in the relationship: from the point of view of an advocate, it's their loved one; from the caregiver's point of view, it's their patient. The emotional investment is much less on the caregiver's part than the advocate's, and occasionally, it's nonexistent.

Wouldn't it be nice if all caregivers, up and down the spectrum of long-term care community staff, considered their roles a *calling, a passion, or a career?* Some do, especially administrators of communities and certified/licensed health professionals. However, those characteristics still don't equal meaningful emotional investment in the individual living in a structured community. There are exceptions, naturally, as the mom observed in the story of the departed caregiver. But still, the caregiver left without any communication.

Some in the long-term care industry will object to these characterizations. Yet our personal experiences say that it's an accurate and credible observation. For many caregivers, it's just a job, sometimes stressful, for which they receive average compensation with the compounded problem of often feeling undervalued. Like all of us, caregivers have struggles outside of the work environment that could impact how care is delivered.

Champions and their loved ones need to recognize this dynamic from the outset. While rules and regulations exist about the quality-of-care residents of assisted living and memory care communities should receive, it's essential to recognize that *individual results will vary.* And we mean the results can and will differ based on the caregiver's mindset.

Here's a somewhat over-the-top example of what we mean: we know a situation where a caregiver in assisted living was exasperated about a resident's difficulty getting out of bed. The resident was unable to roll over due to many illnesses and complications without help and

                    © WatchWorks Management Consulting LLC

said so to the caregiver. In an inexplicable moment of what we assume was a loss of perspective and common sense, the caregiver stated: *Your pain is just in your mind...the problem is you don't want to roll over.* Then, the caregiver stormed out of the resident's room. When we heard this story, we were appalled.

Consider too this distressing incident: a loved one in an independent plus community—a setting that comes with a premium for added assistance—experienced a fall and could not get up. Despite several presses of the emergency call button with no response, the loved one reached out via phone on an Apple Watch. Yet, it still took over fifteen minutes for a caregiver to respond. The resident's advocate arranged a meeting with community management to register concerns. In the session, the champion learned caregivers are trained to treat every assistance request as urgent. Sensible! However, no explanation was offered for why this situation was treated differently.

After this, the same resident experienced a second fall and two presses of the call button; the resident waited almost ten minutes for help to arrive. The advocate requested another meeting and discovered *only one* caregiver was assigned to the 60+ community residents who had paid for this additional emergency service. Despite earlier assertions, community management claimed ten minutes was acceptable, clarifying caregivers would not respond immediately to an alert. They further stated that transferring the resident from independent plus to assisted living would be the best way to manage the resident at a higher cost.

However, we also know stories where the caregiver and community staff were *entirely in the moment,* using their skills and emotional intelligence to help residents. For example, we heard a story about a caregiver who excelled at giving showers and baths to a resident and consistently took great care when manipulating legs and arms, washing hair, and redressing after bathing was done. The loved one and advocate greatly appreciated this caregiver's professional attention.

Or this anecdote about a young caregiver in his early 20s who made it a point every morning before their shift concluded to ensure the resident in his charge had snacks and water within easy reach since they were legally blind and unable to get out of the chair unassisted.

If anything can be learned from this potpourri of examples, *individual results will vary*, and advocates' vigilance is an ongoing requirement.

NOTES

Chapter 3—Job Description for an Advocate/Champion

Pinning down a job description for an advocate/champion has been challenging. There are many possible duties for an advocate to perform. Yet, duties may focus more on one area than another and use different skill sets depending on the community and their loved one's needs. It's a little like writing a job description for life; some things are possible, some are probable, and only a few are certain.

A champion's duties lie squarely upon your loved one's needs. For example, your loved one may be in stable health, i.e., there have been no changes in medications or healthcare protocols, and then suddenly slip and fall, causing injury that restricts mobility. Advocacy looks very different in the first versus second scenario. The first scenario concerns maintaining a routine; the second involves reinventing day-to-day activities like eating, dressing, and bathing. Different knowledge, skills, and abilities are called upon.

Rolling with the punches

This brings us to an advocate's first and foremost requirement: flexibility. Not the ordinary flexibility you may be called upon to exhibit, like a change in the number of people coming to dinner or the need to drive to work using an alternate route. Instead, the type of flexibility required when a wholly unforeseen and possibly tragic event occurs, like a car accident or sudden job loss.

We've wrestled with this and concluded that the colloquial expression rolling with the punches best describes what we mean by flexibility. We can thank the sport of boxing for this helpful phrase. The phrase means avoiding a direct hit (or punch) by having a *strategy*. Boxers may step back or to the side to create a glancing blow versus solid body contact.[16] football players may use a tuck and roll movement to prevent serious injuries when hit.

While we don't much enjoy the thought of a glancing blow as an inevitable outcome, we see the benefit of taking a step back or to the side. Advocates are called upon to use this technique daily. And, to make matters even more interesting, advocates frequently step back and to the side while more than one person is throwing hands at their faces! Being rigid when facing circumstances where the outcome is potentially detrimental to your loved one serves no purpose. Rigidity leads to fewer options and needs to be avoided in favor of flexibility. Now, let's take a crack at an advocate's job description.

General responsibilities of a champion

Advocates are the vital link between loved ones, their families, medical providers, and the long-term care community—whether independent plus, assisted living, or memory care.[17] Advocates' responsibilities include ensuring the needs and preferences of their loved ones are heard, understood, and respected. Champions facilitate effective communication with the community's care team, ensuring changes in their loved one's health and behavior are promptly reviewed and addressed.

Advocates frequently involve themselves in changing their loved ones' care plans, medical treatments, and living arrangements. Champions continuously monitor the quality of care and the community's environment to ensure they align with their loved ones' needs and family expectations.

Advocates play a supportive role in providing emotional encouragement to their loved ones and families, especially when

---

[16] Mayhew, Jeff. "Roll with the Punches," n.d. https://www.weirdfacts.com/en/origin-of-phrases/origin-of-phrases-r/3963-roll-with-the-punches.

[17] Similar statements can be made about the responsibilities of advocates for loved ones in skilled nursing communities. However, we'll continue to focus on assisted living and memory care, comprising about 31,600 communities and 1.2 million beds with over 818,000 residents, representing 2% of the over-65 population in the U.S. as of October 2023. Visit the National Council on Aging website for up-to-date statistics: www.ncoa.org.

changes in the living situation must be made. They also assist family members as a *translator* for the complexities of long-term care. Champions liaise with external healthcare providers, manage administrative tasks related to their loved one's care, and ensure legal and financial matters are handled correctly and promptly.

In memory care communities, champions play a heightened role along the full spectrum of care requirements due to their loved ones' incapacity. The responsibilities are generally the same as cited above, but loved ones are much less active in their healthcare decisions.

Skills, knowledge, and abilities of a champion

Advocates must possess specific skills, including effective communication, persistence, tenacity, problem-solving, negotiating, organizing and documenting, curiosity, and learning agility. Champions must understand relationship management with caregivers, providers, community staff, and administrators by applying high levels of emotional intelligence, including empathy, social skills, self-awareness, and self-regulation amid potentially chaotic and exceptional circumstances.

To make intelligent recommendations, advocates should familiarize themselves with existing long-term care bodies of knowledge to correctly interpret the contexts in which the daily activities of loved ones will play out. Below are examples of high-value knowledge areas for champions:

1) **Medical**—Understanding their loved one's medical conditions, treatments, medications (including potential side effects), and commonly used terminology.
2) **Insurance and healthcare financing**—Understanding how health insurance works, the role of Medicare and Medicaid, Advantage Plans and Supplemental Plans, coverage details (including deductibles and co-pays), and the expert referral process.

3) **Gerontology**—Understanding the biological, psychological, cognitive, cultural, and social aspects of aging.[18]
4) **Important documents**—Long-term care insurance provisions, federal and state laws, and regulations governing assisted living and memory care communities, including leases, resident handbooks, standards of care, and residents' rights.
5) **Legal knowledge**—Understanding the terminology and appointment provisions of a power of attorney, healthcare directive, guardianship, and trusts/wills.

Duties and tasks of a champion

- Reading, understanding, and interpreting leases, agreements, and community handbooks, especially about daily routines and protocols.
- Becoming familiar with services available in the community, such as in-house physical, occupational, and speech therapy, medication management, and medical care. Note: third-party contractors frequently deliver services.
- Requesting and attending formal and informal meetings with community staff to facilitate the monitoring of care delivery.
- Coordinating medical treatments inside and outside the community, including primary care physicians and specialists, pharmacists, dentists, ophthalmologists, audiologists, PT/OT therapists, podiatrists, and mental health professionals.
- Building and maintaining solid relationships with those involved in delivering care with a particular focus on staff members who directly interact with a loved one.
- Making suggestions and recommendations on adjustments to a loved one's care plan, following up personally and in writing, as needed, to implement changes.
- Ensuring superior care for a loved one, particularly those unusually vulnerable due to physical, cognitive, speech, memory, or other issues.

---

[18] Wikipedia contributors. "Gerontology." Wikipedia, January 5, 2024. https://en.wikipedia.org/wiki/Gerontology.

- Providing insights to caregivers about a loved one's personal & family history, preferences, special needs, concerns, and limitations.
- Providing emotional support to a loved one, building trust, and adhering to agreed-upon boundaries.
- Visiting/checking in with a loved one regularly, including in-person, via phone calls, Facetime, or online visual tools like Teams and Zoom.
- Communicating with other family members about a loved one's health, well-being, and changing needs.
- Shopping for personal care items, clothing, toiletries, snacks, and reading material.
- Documenting unresolved community concerns, maintaining personal copies, and providing copies to community administrators.
- Ensuring financial obligations are met on time and monitoring community fees for approved add-on services or unexpected charges.

Primary relationships of a champion

Below is a list of the relationships advocates must maintain to be effective. Included is one fundamental expectation from individuals in each group.

1) **Family members and friends**—Maintain open lines of communication with the champion and pass along any new information.
2) **Management staff**—Be transparent regarding policies, procedures, and changes within the community.
3) **Financial and accounting staff**—Maintain accurate billing and explain and justify all charges.
4) **Healthcare staff/aides**—Provide competent, compassionate, and individualized care according to the documented healthcare plan.
5) **Housekeeping staff**—Ensure a clean, safe, and comfortable living environment.

6) **Dietitians, chefs, cooks, and servers**—Create nutritious meals that accommodate dietary restrictions and align with personal tastes and health needs.

7) **Physicians, specialists, podiatrists, nurse practitioners, and nurses**—Provide prompt medical care, including regular assessments.

8) **Physical, occupational, and speech therapists**—Ensure fit-for-purpose, consistent therapy programs to maintain or improve quality of life.

9) **Fellow community residents and family members**—Continuously promote community and mutual respect, fostering a consistently supportive environment.

10) **Other service providers, such as mobile X-ray technicians and hairstylists**—Provide professional, courteous services that accommodate schedules and preferences.

There are other relationships you will need to be attentive to—and from whom you should receive high-quality service. These include Medicare, Medicaid, and insurance company representatives. In all the enumerated relationships, champions may find the need to explain their expectations. We agree and hope you will find it within yourself to be patient and agreeable in those moments.

Keep calm and carry on—you will grow into a champion

Have you ever applied for a new job with a new employer and been confronted with a job description that *partly but not wholly* describes you? We have, which sometimes prevents us from considering the job opportunity in detail. You may have thought *I didn't know how to do this, or I'm sure others who are more qualified than me will apply.* Both of these and other reactions are valid.

But recall, nearly all job descriptions are *aspirational.* This means employers ask for precisely what they want, knowing most applicants will miss one or more skill sets or need more experience in specifically enumerated duties. Both of us had hiring authority in our past professional positions. We came to expect applicants would have only some of the necessary skills or experiences, and in the end, we needed to weigh other factors.

The most important quality we've found overall is a *positive mindset.* In our experience, if a candidate had most of the skills and knowledge, we relied more heavily on assessing their positivity, enthusiasm, and *can-do* attitude. Mindset plus the willingness to learn and adapt goes a long way to filling in any gaps on the candidate's resume.

Champions with the proper mindset, a willingness to learn, change, and grow—plus a dose of humility—will achieve what they need for their loved ones. We believe giving up and going with the flow will not work. Constant effort is required. Feeling tired and daunted by this? We are, too, but it's incalculably worth the effort. We consider it a privilege and an honor to be champions for our mothers.

NOTES

Chapter 4—Effective Communication Skills

Basics of effective communication skills

Effective communication involves being clear and concise, expressing concerns with appropriate passion, asking penetrating questions, and listening. Building ties with caregivers, including managers, doctors, nurses, and aides, is essential. Creating and maintaining positive relationships will help achieve the best care possible.

A manager confided in us, saying that family members had yelled at and belittled them over resident care issues. They dreaded these emotional encounters. They confessed they had built a thick skin, causing them to hesitate, even in obvious and urgent situations.

This is an excellent example of the need for champions to demonstrate practical and considerate communication skills. It's also a sure sign that caring for a loved one can be impeded due to poor interactions.

Improving your communication skills

- **Prepare in advance**—Verify you'll be speaking to the right person. Have your facts straight. Write down the plan of what you will say and do.
- **Be clear and concise**—Focus on the problem, not past issues or free-floating worries. Avoid family storytelling. Recognize that fewer words lead to faster understanding.
- **Be respectful**—Use personal names when you can. Point to the problem and not the individual. Honor the person's role in the life of your loved one.
- **Ask thoughtful questions**—Refrain from declarative statements. Formulate open-ended queries versus yes/no. Avoid judgmental words and phrases.

- **Maintain emotional balance**—Show your passion, but don't yell or shout. Recognize that the other person's feelings about your loved one will never equal yours.
- **Listen with purpose**—Stop talking after you ask a question to allow for an answer. Paraphrase back what you heard. Don't speak over the other person.
- **Show up confidently**—Act as though you belong. Develop a compelling presence. Pitch your voice so the other person doesn't need to strain to hear you.
- **Adjust conversational focus**—Avoid using *you/your/they/them* statements and instead use *we/us/our* to create a sense of teamwork and a greater emphasis on your loved one.

Sandwich feedback method

When you have little time to prepare for an interaction, a champion could use the sandwich feedback method to improve communications. This three-step process helps to ensure the conversation is positive while allowing you to offer suggestions on improvements and ask potentially challenging questions.

1) Start with a positive, confirming comment—Compliment the person for something they did well and express appreciation for their continued efforts. Set a supportive tone.

2) Offer feedback, make constructive suggestions, or ask thoughtful questions—Clarify the new, beneficial behavior. Be specific and fact-based. Empathetically focus on the caregiver's actions at work.

3) End with a positive, hopeful comment—Express encouragement and show confidence in the caregiver's abilities. (While you could reiterate your conversational opening, we suggest you finish with something new/different.)

Adam Molinsky wrote a thought-provoking article you might find instructive on becoming proficient in the sandwich feedback method—*Reinventing the Feedback Sandwich: 5 Different Ways.*[19]

---

[19] Molinsky, Andy. "Reinventing the Feedback Sandwich - 5 Different Ways - Andy Molinsky." Andy Molinsky, June 23, 2016. https://www.andymolinsky.com/reinventing-feedback-sandwich-5-different-ways/.

Scenario—effective communication

It's 1:00 p.m., you just arrived at your grandmother's community, and you learn she missed lunch and is hungry.

One Way	A Better Way
Champion: My grandmother told me she didn't eat lunch today. That should never happen! She needs to eat and can't get to the dining room alone. **Caregiver:** We checked in with every resident today and asked them if they wanted lunch, your grandmother included. She said she wasn't hungry. **Champion:** That's not what she told me; this has happened before. You need to get her something to eat. **Caregiver:** Lunch is over, and dinner isn't for another two hours. There's nothing I can do about it since the kitchen is closed. **Champion:** That's not good enough. Who is your on-duty supervisor? I need to talk to them and straighten this out. **Caregiver:** I'll try to find her. Give me a few minutes. **Champion:** We need to get food to my grandmother immediately!	**Champion:** Hello Tina, I'm not sure if you remember me. I'm Joseph, Helen Jones's grandson. How are you doing today? Busy as usual? **Caregiver:** It's another hectic day, but I'm making it through. Thanks for asking. What can I do for you? **Champion:** I'm wondering how Helen is doing with meals—has she had much appetite today? **Caregiver:** Not really. When we went to get her for lunch, Helen said she wasn't hungry. We even tried again later. **Champion:** Oh, I see. You know, Helen may have changed her mind about being hungry. Another 90 minutes have passed since you asked her. I think Helen's hungry. What do you suggest? **Caregiver:** The kitchen is closed. But would she eat a snack to hold her until dinner? **Champion:** That'd be great. What do you have? Almost anything could work.

While it may seem the dialog on the left above wouldn't happen, in our experience, it can and does. Advocates are as fallible as the next person and can assume too much, jump to a conclusion, or engage in an unfortunate interaction with a caregiver. No doubt the champion in the scenario has the best interests of their loved one in mind. Yet the *prickly-pear* approach fails to hit the mark and generally slows the response to the problem, i.e., Grandma is hungry.

The *A Better Way* possibility, shown on the right in the table, begins on the human side by letting the staff member know who you represent and then asking a non-confrontational question: *I'm wondering how my grandmother has been doing today with meals.* There is no assumption nor an accusatory tone. Such an approach will get results much faster, plus maintain or even improve the relationship.

Note also that the champion used the loved one's name rather than just the personal relationship identification. Why is this important? Because caregivers address residents using their proper names and aren't always able to keep all the relatives straight in their minds.

This is our final thought on effective communication from Artell's recent book, *Engage.Coach.Develop: Building Strong Relationships that Drive Individual and Team Performance:*

Always begin on the human side. Get to know the person in context. Be appropriately curious, and ensure you listen to what the person says.[20]

---

[20] Smith, Artell. *Engage.Coach.Develop: Building Strong Relationships That Drive Individual and Team Performance.* iUniverse, 2023. Page 14.

NOTES

Chapter 5—Persistence and Tenacity Skills

Basics of persistence and tenacity skills

Quoting Benjamin Franklin: *Energy and persistence conquer all things.*[21] We like Franklin's thought since it applies to the role of an advocate and champion. Few good things will happen in the life of your loved one without a heavy dose of persistence and tenacity.

You'll encounter situations where you may think it's better to turn right while your loved one wants to turn left. This is natural. Champions first perceive situations based on their experiences and, second, based on their loved ones. We must remind ourselves daily that being an advocate is not about us! We may think we know what's best, but sometimes we don't.

Advocates need to know their loved ones well enough to understand and verbalize their wishes, choices, care needs, desired involvement in the community, etc. A champion should fulfill their loved one's wishes to the best of their abilities. This means consistently confirming their desires, which is your first objective.

For example, we know an advocate whose loved one enjoyed jigsaw puzzles. The community had two places with jigsaw puzzles where residents could sit, talk, and work on puzzles. When the advocate suggested working on puzzles might be good and pushed in that direction, the loved one responded that doing so left no personal time for phone calls, daily therapeutic appointments, going to meals, etc. The advocate learned something important by listening closely to their loved one.

We know of another champion who struggled to understand why their loved one received a request to move rooms. After receiving no

---

[21] BrainyQuote. "Benjamin Franklin Quotes," n.d.
   https://www.brainyquote.com/quotes/benjamin_franklin_378118.

answers to their questions, the advocate convened the care team to discuss. In the meeting, the advocate learned only one caregiver wanted the room changed but had no credible reason. The community withdrew the request. Without the advocate's efforts, the move would have occurred, causing disruption and emotional trauma for the loved one.

Improving your persistence and tenacity skills

- **Focus on the desired outcome**—Be clear on your goals and objectives before you engage with loved ones, family members, or caregivers. If possible, reason out first what matters most.
- **Compress your emotions**— Recognize your persistence may elicit emotional responses from others. Tightly contain and manage your emotions to avoid instantly regretted statements.
- *One-and-done* **may not work**—Coach yourself to accept multiple interactions may be needed to resolve an issue. Attempting to address problems too quickly can fray relationships.
- **Listen to other residents' and advocates' stories**—Leverage the experiences of community residents and fellow champions. Acknowledge the possibility that you may not be correct. Keep your mind open to counsel.
- **Step away when needed**—Seek out a quiet place, contemplate your past and future approaches, and generate alternative scenarios. *Sleep on it*, a proven technique for piercing through cloudy logic.

Scenario—persistence and tenacity

In a conversation with the on-duty nurse, you discover that a medication prescribed for your mother in a memory care community is not being regularly administered because it was incorrectly marked as *requested by the resident.*

One Way	A Better Way
Champion: The doctor prescribed that medication almost a week ago; why isn't it being administered? **Nurse:** This med is marked *requested by the resident,* so we can't do otherwise. **Champion:** That makes no sense, don't you see? My mother would never request the medication. She can't make her own decisions. She has a chronic condition. **Nurse:** We can't force residents to take medication if they don't want to. That's against our policy. **Champion:** I'm not asking you to force her to take the medication; I'm asking why it hasn't been included in her regular schedule. She would never ask. **Nurse:** You'll have to talk with her doctor. I can't make a change because you tell me to. I administer the meds based on the instructions. **Champion:** So, you're saying that's it? You won't help me? This is a medication my mother needs! **Nurse:** Until we get new instructions, it's out of my hands. **Champion:** Then I will have to handle it myself. I will have a lot more to say after this is dealt with.	**Champion:** If I remember correctly, my mother's doctor prescribed the new medication about a week ago. **Nurse:** Yes, that's right. But your mother hasn't requested it yet, so I don't have any record of it. **Champion:** I understand. Are there other medications marked like that? It seems unusual, given my mother's condition. **Nurse:** No, that's the only one. **Champion:** In your judgment, do you think there was an error? **Nurse:** I suppose. It's not *impossible.* **Champion:** That's what I am thinking, too. What would be the best way to confirm? **Nurse:** I could put a call into the doctor's office. I can't do it right now, though, since I'm making the rounds with medications. **Champion:** Makes sense. How about this? I will call and check in with you in a couple of hours. Would that work? **Nurse:** I will be here, but I don't always hear back from doctors' offices quickly! **Champion:** I understand. Let's see what we can do!

The issue in the scenario above is among the most serious we can think of. There are worse, to be sure, especially in emergencies when a health crisis occurs. However, failure to administer timely medications can cause serious negative medical consequences for your loved one. A level of persistence and tenacity is required to resolve such issues quickly.

It may be helpful to remember a busy caregiver, like a nurse, licensed practical nurse, or medical assistant, has many residents to keep track of. Forgetting details about who receives which medication and at what time is relatively commonplace. This is why such heavy reliance on written prescription instructions should happen. Deviating from prescribed routines creates liability for the community and the loved one and is also a cause for concern for advocates.

Approaching the scenario from *A Better Way* perspective has at least four advantages: 1) The champion starts with a routine question and follows up with a second; 2) No *statements* are made; 3) The champion appeals to the caregiver's expertise by using the phrase *in your judgment*; and 4) The champion creates an intentional timeline for the next steps.

Referring to our list of essential behaviors for persistence and tenacity, the Champion demonstrates clarity on the desired outcome throughout the interaction, avoids emotional outbursts, and recognizes minimally that a second interaction is needed. The chances of faster success using an approach like this are high.

Dale Carnegie said:

Flaming enthusiasm, backed up by horse sense and persistence, is the quality that most frequently makes for success.[22]

---

[22] Conlow, Rick, and Rick Conlow. 2022. "50 Persistence Quotes That Inspire & Motivate | Rick Conlow." Rick Conlow. December 11, 2022. https://rickconlow.com/50-persistence-quotes-inspire-motivate/.

NOTES

Chapter 6—Problem-Solving and Negotiating Skills

Basics of problem-solving and negotiating skills

If your only tool is a hammer, everything looks like a nail, said Abraham Maslow or Mark Twain.[23] Researchers of famous quotes aren't quite sure. However, the quote's meaning is transparent and pertains to our discussion of problem-solving and negotiating.

A problem-solving and negotiating skill set definition may help identify, analyze, and effectively resolve challenges or conflicts mutually agreed upon by all parties involved. Components of this skill set include critical thinking, root cause analysis, creativity, and solid interpersonal behaviors. Becoming proficient in this skill set often involves viewing issues from multiple perspectives and communicating clearly and persuasively. When done well, relationships will grow and strengthen.

In our experience, people tend to solve problems using their current and comfortable areas of expertise rather than branching out and trying different techniques. This is expected, but it does leave things *on the table.* The work of a loved one's champion requires many different approaches to solving problems.

For example, we've noted a tendency for assisted living and memory care communities to rush to one particular answer in a specific situation, namely when a decision must be made to transport a loved one who has fallen to the hospital emergency room. Sometimes, this decision is made so quickly that 9-1-1 or an ambulance is called moments after an incident happens without any attempt to evaluate.

---

[23] Quoteresearch. "If Your Only Tool Is a Hammer Then Every Problem Looks like a Nail – Quote Investigator®," May 8, 2014.
   https://quoteinvestigator.com/2014/05/08/hammer-nail/.

We agree that the 9-1-1 ambulance transport option is a possible solution for a loved one who falls. However, we disagree with the *rush to judgment* that typically precedes calling an ambulance. Wouldn't it be better to evaluate the facts first? This is *definitely* where an advocate comes in. A call should first be made to the person who holds the medical POA. Transport to an emergency room is a jarring experience for seniors and should be used only after applying a criterion-referenced decision-making process.[24]

Improving your problem-solving and negotiating skills

- **Formulate a best-case problem description**—Describe the situation using neutral language. Remove emotion from your report. Avoid mentioning the names of individuals other than your loved one's name.[25]
- **Self-interrogate to generate root cause**—Ask yourself simple questions to create possible reasons for the problem. Use *what, where, when, why, and how* techniques. Write down the answers.
- **Consider how others could react**—Assume your point of view is only one of several alternatives. Admit you may be wrong in your assessment. Ask other champions for their thoughts.
- **Brainstorm creative solutions**—List possible ways the situation could be resolved or avoided in the future. Devote a few minutes of focused concentration to this exercise. Prioritize your list, asking yourself *what the path of least resistance is.*
- **Determine flexibility limits**—Consider which elements of your preferred solution could be given up or traded for another. Move toward an entirely acceptable outcome for all parties. Recalling your loved one's needs is more important than your opinions.

---

[24] There has been extensive research on whether to transport after a fall. You may want to explore this topic. A 2017 National Institutes of Health study may help: "Transport to the Emergency Department for Assisted Living Residents Who Fall." *Annals of Internal Medicine* 168, no. 3 (December 12, 2017): 1–26. https://doi.org/10.7326/p17-9051.

[25] For tips on selectively including your emotions in conversations, see Chapter 4, Essential Skills for Champions—Emotional Intelligence, the section labeled *When emotional intelligence includes a display of emotion.*

Scenario—problem-solving and negotiating

Your great-aunt told you today that she hasn't had a shower or bath in over a week and worries she's been forgotten.

One Way	A Better Way
Champion—My great-aunt informed me she hasn't had a shower in a week, and I need to know why. Did Nadine forget? **Caregiver**—I can tell your great-aunt was scheduled for Thursday afternoon, but she said she wasn't up to it. That's the note another caregiver put in the file. **Champion**—OK, but why didn't someone return later to try again? That would have been the right thing to do! **Caregiver**—Because other residents are scheduled for their showers, putting her back on the schedule would have delayed someone else. **Champion**—Are you telling me you don't have enough staff to accommodate a simple shower schedule change? What on earth are we paying for? **Caregiver**—I'm only here Tuesday through Friday, so I can't tell you what happened the other days. You'll have to talk to someone who was here Friday through Monday to determine why she wasn't worked in. **Champion**—Today is Tuesday, so my great-aunt must wait two more days for her shower? **Caregiver**—Yes, that's right.	**Champion**—Hi Dana, I'm Joe, and Carol is my great-aunt. I have a quick question. Do you have time now? **Caregiver**—Yes, lunch service doesn't start for another 20 minutes. What can I help you with? **Champion**—Carol is worried about her weekly shower and wondering when she could be worked into the schedule. I think she's a little uncomfortable. **Caregiver**—That's going to be difficult. Her normal day is Thursday. I doubt we can do anything for Carol today. Another resident would need to be shifted. **Champion**—I'm thinking there are a few good reasons she missed her normal day. Regardless, she didn't realize she'd have to wait a week. **Caregiver**—Carol doesn't always enjoy her showers. She's on a different person's schedule who is not here today. **Champion**—I understand. Carol has good days and bad days. Could we move it up just one day? It's Tuesday, so what about tomorrow after breakfast? Or even afternoon? I need your help to figure it out. **Caregiver**—I can't make any promises, but I understand the situation better now. Let me see what I can do.

An important takeaway from the scenario above is it's tough to assemble all the facts and decide which are most important. The loved one had some information; the caregiver had a second set of data points; the champion had a third, including their opinion. What's vital in the scenario is the loved one needs a shower! The champion must put all other considerations aside to achieve the desired outcome, including their sense of *what's logical.*

Picking up on a theme in a previous chapter, staffing *still* needs to be solved for long-term care communities. Among community staff, the caregivers are the least able to influence this. Pointing fingers or declaring more people should be available to provide services is a dead end. Most caregivers agree more staff is needed.

Starting a discussion with a couple of non-confrontational questions is a best practice. Admitting their loved one could have rejected the shower for various reasons is also a good tactic for the champion. Placing options in front of the caregiver and enlisting their help to solve the problem *together* is likewise essential.

Last thought: As you read the column on the right above, you may conclude that there are too many words, and you would never phrase your conversation as we suggest. Depending on your mindset, we understand and offer an alternative that could work.

Champion—I see you're busy, and I don't want to take up your time. But I have a question.

Caregiver—Yes?

Champion—Carol has been suffering a bit since she missed her shower last week. It's nobody's fault, but here we are! Is there a way to work her into the schedule?

Caregiver—Working her into the schedule today will be hard.

Champion—I understand. To give time to adjust, what about tomorrow morning or afternoon? Even a day sooner would make a difference.

Caregiver—I'll see what I can do.

Champion—I appreciate your help. I know this is above and beyond.

A more abbreviated conversation between the champion and caregiver is possible because the champion thought through the problem and the most likely solution to meet the need. The champion also did not demand an explanation of *why* her great-aunt was skipped. Pursuing this route cuts the total number of words by half. Less can be better!

Most caregivers appreciate the advocate getting to the point quickly. However, in our experience, it's sometimes difficult to reach the caregiver and stand still long enough to have a conversation, even a short one. This is symptomatic of the more significant staffing issues in long-term care communities.

Problems beg to be solved! Don't disappoint them.

NOTES

Chapter 7—Organization and Documentation Skills

Basics of organization and documentation skills

In Chapter 3, we presented a job description for an advocate, including general responsibilities, skills/knowledge/abilities, and duties/tasks to be performed regularly. We also suggested diligent champions maintain a baker's dozen crucial relationships on their loved one's behalf. We turn to those vital relationships in our description of the organization and documentation skill set.

We've observed the paperwork accountability of champions to be very challenging to some. Occasionally, we're overwhelmed with a seemingly endless stream of electronic or hardcopy documents: the overlapping arrays of applications, leases, resident handbooks, community policies, processes, terms & conditions, timelines/schedules, invoices, benefits statements, banking information, insurance forms, etc., are genuinely bewildering and require deep focus.

Organization and documentation refer to the ability to systematically arrange and manage tasks, information, and documents, ensuring they're easily accessible and trackable. Lack of attention to detail is a significant speed bump on the journey with your loved one. It's seductive to think this is just one piece of paper; how much could it matter, OR this is only one line item in the care plan...I can trust caregivers to focus on the big picture. We wish this were true since it would greatly simplify the lives of champions.

Staying on top of the many moving parts will give you confidence. Over time, you'll know more about your loved one than anyone they associate with. Most people and organizations with an ongoing relationship cannot see all the moving parts and frequently don't care to exert the effort. Assisted living and memory care communities are attentive to their cash flow and bottom line. This is true of nearly all the care communities you'll encounter, even those who describe themselves as non-profit. Your advocacy power goes beyond simply having a POA on file; it's highly related to your archive of relevant knowledge.

Improving your organization and documentation skills

- **Take inventory**—Locate all the electronic and physical documentation related to your loved one's situation, going back at least 24 months, and gather it together. Then, determine the *place(s)* to store the documentation, likely a combination of electronic and paper files.
- **Determine filing and retrieval approach**—Decide how you'll logically and quickly fetch information based on your preferences; organize documentation accordingly.[26]
- **Leverage technology's benefits**—Create shortcuts to critical documents and other information by investing in one of several mobile applications designed to keep track of everything[27]; minimally use your phone to take pictures of key documents and store them on your phone and in email account folders.
- **Become a list maker**—Use old-fashioned paper and pen to write down tasks that need to be accomplished, supplies to be purchased, and people who need to be contacted; send yourself text messages or emails; use the *task list* feature available in your email app.
- **Seek others for help**—Connect with family members/friends and ask for assistance locating and organizing critical information; find a professional organizer using Google or another online search engine and schedule an appointment.

---

[26] There are many possible file-and-retrieve approaches. We've found it helpful to organize based on the discreet relationships you manage on behalf of your loved one. Refer to our list of typical relationships in Chapter 3.

[27] We recommend a relatively new mobile application called *Prisidio,* developed by Age Tech Collaborative, a start-up company in partnership with the American Association of Retired Persons (AARP). For details about *Prisidio,* check out their website at www.prisid.io.

Documentation priorities

We frequently refer to a few documents and recommend keeping them handy. Start here in your efforts to become better organized. You can create a personal notebook or store these items in an expandable folder.

1) ID cards for Medicare, Medicaid, Advantage, and Supplemental insurance plans, including vision, dental, hearing, and prescription drugs.
2) List of medications taken with dosage amounts and times.
3) Power-of-attorney documents showing your loved one's agents.
4) Do Not Resuscitate (DNR) documents, if any.
5) Provider and community contact emails and phone numbers, including administrators, physicians, therapists, pharmacists, dentists, etc.
6) Community-provided documents. For example, applications, leases, handbooks, community policies, etc.
7) Electronic medical records.
8) Hard copies of emails you send on essential topics.

Note: If you're dealing with care issues, meeting face-to-face and writing down everything is essential. Record who attended, the problem, the better ways to solve it, and what everyone agreed on. Share the notes with everyone at the meeting, including community leadership, even if they did not attend. Ask for confirmation of receipt. If problems persist, these notes might help later. Also, keep a paper copy safe.

Scenario—Organization and documentation

You're in the hospital emergency room with your sister, who lives in a memory care community. You're in the middle of the registration process.

One Way	A Better Way
Registration Clerk—Hello, my job here is to register your loved one for emergency room services and possible admission to the hospital if needed. What is your relationship with the patient? **Champion**—I'm Janet's sister, and I have a POA for healthcare decisions. Do you need a copy of the POA? I don't have it with me right now. **Registration Clerk**—We can collect that later; I can give you the email to send the POA. What's your sister's full name, address, and phone number? **Champion**—Janet Elizabeth Cooper, whose address Is 42 Maple Street in town. She has no phone number, but I can give you mine. **Registration Clerk**—Very good. Does Ms. Cooper live at that address? **Champion**—Oh no, sorry. She's in a memory care living community. **Registration Clerk**—Can you look up the address? I'll also need your sister's health insurance and med list. **Champion**—I'm sorry, I don't have any of that handy; I will need to call someone.	**Registration Clerk**—Hello, my job here is to register your loved one for emergency room services and possible admission to the hospital if needed. What is your relationship with the patient? **Champion**—I'm Janet's sister, an authorized POA for healthcare decisions. I have an electronic copy of the POA if you need it. I also have information about her Medicare Supplemental Insurance Plan. **Registration Clerk**—That's great! I'll take all that information, and also, I'll need her medication list. Have you ever been to this hospital before? **Champion**—No, this is Janet's first time here. I have the med list. **Registration Clerk**—Let's get started.

Enough said

The above scenario speaks for itself. There's nothing more uncomfortable than being authorized to speak for your loved one but unable to produce documentation or provide essential information. Functionaries at all healthcare facilities, from assisted living, memory care communities, urgent care clinics, doctor's offices, pharmacies, and hospitals, all need the same basic information. Their confidence in you as a valid advocate will increase significantly *if you produce the goods.*

If you lack all the correct information, you need at least the contact details of someone who does, including those from the assisted living or memory care community. Upon admission to the community, they would have collected the data requested by the registration clerk in the preceding example. Remember, too, the better your relationship with community staff, the easier it will be when urgent moments arrive in your loved one's life.

We recently had an opportunity to *practice what we preach* regarding this skill set. A loved one was brought to the hospital emergency room by ambulance. The community had done its part by handing over necessary paperwork, like recent test results and Medicare information. But in the rush of calling an ambulance and getting the loved one on board, the paperwork mistakenly omitted information about Supplemental Insurance. A casual question to the registration clerk revealed the problem. Luckily, we had taken pictures of the ID cards, called them up immediately from our photo library, and relayed the details. What a mess that would have been!

NOTES

Chapter 8—Curiosity and Learning Agility Skills

Basics of curiosity and learning agility skills

Human curiosity is fundamental to our nature. It's rooted in the evolutionary and cognitive development of the species. Curiosity leads to exploration and learning. Ancient humans survived harsh environments by asking two simple questions: why? And what if? They learned from their surroundings and tried new ways to hunt and gather food. This improved their chances of survival. [28]

A 2014 study published In *Neuron* reported curiosity activates the brain's reward centers, prompting a sense of satisfaction and a desire to learn more. Curiosity creates a positive state of mind, stimulates our desire to learn, and releases dopamine. That's a good deal all the way around! [29]

Our primary purpose in *Champion's Needed* is to help advocates make a positive difference in their loved one's lives. Curiosity and its follow-on desire to learn do just that. Curiosity can be your superpower. We sincerely mean this. At the outset, champions must admit applying their logic and experience to issues only goes so far. We both know people who apply only what they know right now to situations where brand-new information is needed.

If advocates use open-ended questions, they'll gain knowledge in a socially acceptable fashion, enabling immediate application. Open-

---

[28] Gruber, Matthias J., Bernard D. Gelman, and Charan Ranganath. "States of Curiosity Modulate Hippocampus-Dependent Learning via the Dopaminergic Circuit." *Neuron* 84, no. 2 (October 1, 2014): 486–96. https://doi.org/10.1016/j.neuron.2014.08.060.

[29] See this article for a summary of the study published in *Neuron:* EurekAlert! "How Curiosity Changes the Brain to Enhance Learning," October 2, 2014. https://www.eurekalert.org/news-releases/500062.

ended questioning techniques aren't admired as much as they should be.

Examples of open-ended questions

1) What are your ideas for encouraging my loved one to socialize more?
2) What's your evaluation of my loved one's appetite?
3) What do you see daily in my loved one's ability to use their walker or wheelchair?
4) How is my loved one managing in small group settings?
5) What do you think is causing my loved one's anxiety about leaving their room?
6) What are your observations on how my loved one is faring with their new medication?
7) How are you fulfilling this service described in my loved one's care plan?

The questions above are all lead-ins to longer, more robust conversations. Honoring the expertise of those in contact with your loved one creates feelings of both respect and comfort. Champions are not present in the entire lives of their loved ones and must always recall that *what happens when you are not there* is more important than *what happens in your presence*. Relying on your innate curiosity and a thoughtful questioning strategy will result in more positive experiences for your loved one.

Since curiosity is only half of this skill set, let's now turn to *learning agility.*

A straightforward approach for this skill set is to imagine your future actions when information is provided to you as an outcome of your curiosity. Does the new information spur you to act? Or does it merely give you an opening to verbalize a statement based on your preconceived notions? If the latter, then we've done a poor job as authors!

Learning agility is quickly comprehending and adapting to new information, changing environments, and recent experiences.

Someone who possesses learning agility embraces the unknown and works toward understanding.[30] It's tightly linked to the neuroplasticity of our brains, which typically diminishes as we get older. High neuroplasticity allows the brain to reorganize itself, allowing for cognitive growth.

If you have heard someone described as a *quick learner,* you already know what learning agility *means.* We believe this skill set is not about intelligence quotient or IQ. Personalizing will be about your ability to accept the situations presented to you without judgment—ask questions to learn more, evaluate options, and acquire new skills to survive and thrive.

Improving your curiosity and learning agility skills

- **Study and read up**—Surf the internet for new topics to benefit you and your loved one. Use artificial intelligence programs and interrogate them on areas of knowledge that might be beneficial. Dedicate 2-3 times each week to these efforts.
- **Rehearse beforehand**—Think of, then practice, the questions you'll ask and imagine the responses you could receive. Consider possible *answers to the reactions* and modify your questions accordingly.
- **Seek feedback and reflect**—Ask others for input on ideas. Slow down to evaluate your conversation and how people around you reacted. Look back on prior interactions and contemplate *a better way.*
- **Experiment and take measured risks**—Seek out new activities that challenge and potentially make you uncomfortable. Try out new behaviors to determine what is practical. Discuss differences with others in ways that lead to learning and change.

---

[30] Hoff, David F., and W. Warner Burke. *Learning Agility,* 2017.

Scenario—curiosity and learning agility

You're walking into your uncle's memory care community to visit him. Upon entering, you're pulled aside by the on-site physical and occupational therapist, who is asserting your uncle should begin as soon as possible for his and other residents' well-being.

One Way	A Better Way
PT/OT Therapist—Hello, Ms. Jones. I need to talk to you about your uncle. I've done a second evaluation on him, and I feel now is the right time to start PT/OT.	**PT/OT Therapist**—Hello, Ms. Jones. I need to talk to you about your uncle. I've done a second evaluation on him, and I feel now is the right time to start PT/OT.
Champion—Slow down a bit, ok? Who authorized a second evaluation? A therapist already said it wasn't needed. I don't remember her name or yours.	**Champion**—Um, yes, hello. Sorry, my mind was somewhere else, um, Matt. Are we talking about Bennett Brown?
PT/OT Therapist—My name's Matt. We've been introduced before. It's routine to do follow-up evaluations, given your uncle nearly fell yesterday; plus, he said it was okay with him.	**PT/OT Therapist**—Yes. Your uncle should be seeing someone on my staff at least weekly, given he almost fell yesterday.
Champion—I would've expected a phone call before anything was done, especially if it was a serious event.	**Champion**—Oh! I didn't know. A fall is very concerning, Matt. I agree with you. I worry about that a lot for my uncle. What can you tell me about the incident?
PT/OT Therapist—No, this event wasn't serious; that's my point. If the aides hadn't been nearby, your uncle would have hit the ground. Who knows how bad it could have been?	**PT/OT Therapist**—I didn't see it personally, but two aides told me it was a close call. They said he was getting up from his chair when it happened. I'm concerned it's only a matter of time before he hurts himself.
Champion—Well, thank heavens he didn't fall! I'm on my way now to see my uncle. I'll let you know what we decide tomorrow or the next day. Thanks.	**Champion**—I understand, Matt. If you have time, I'm going to see my uncle right now...What types of therapy do you want to focus on? Let's discuss this while we walk together to his room.

The champion's information-gathering technique in *A Better Way* above is subtle but very effective. In addition, the champion exercised emotional intelligence during the interaction. While potentially perceived as abrupt, the PT/OT Therapist can also be viewed as simply fulfilling the duties of his job. Specifically, a resident had a near-miss fall; loss of balance was likely the culprit, and an evaluation was needed. We agree; however, their *bedside manner* could be improved.

The champion's two beneficial questions were these: 1) What can you tell me about the incident? And 2) What types of therapy do you want to focus on?

It's true. The champion should be concerned they were not informed about the *near-miss fall*. And it's natural they wonder about the *follow-up evaluation.* Yet, those issues are secondary, given the repercussions of a loved one falling. The Centers for Disease Control and Prevention (CDC) has reported one in four senior adults falls each year and that in 2021, nearly 39,000 seniors aged 65 and older *died* from preventable falls. Another 2.9 million seniors were treated in emergency rooms in the same year.[31]

Curiosity can be your superpower, along with the benefit of learning something new. To achieve success in developing these skills, you must exhibit a willingness to set aside, at least temporarily, any preconceived notions of how the world works based on prior experiences and established mindsets.[32]

---

[31] Injury Facts. "Older Adult Falls - Injury Facts," November 6, 2023.
https://injuryfacts.nsc.org/home-and-community/safety-topics/older-adult-falls/#:~:text=Safety%20Topics,-Older%20Adult%20Falls&text=According%20to%20the%20Centers%20for,were%20treated%20in%20emergency%20departments.
[32] Smith, Artell. *Engage.Coach.Develop: Building Strong Relationships That Drive Individual and Team* Performance. iUniverse, 2023. Page 46

NOTES

Chapter 9—Emotional Intelligence Skills

Basics of emotional intelligence skills

If we were to lead a brainstorming session with the question--*what are an advocate's most essential skills?—we* would want someone to suggest the skills and behaviors associated with emotional intelligence. Dr. Dan Goleman went a long way toward explaining emotional intelligence in his path-clearing book *Emotional Intelligence: Why It Can Matter More than IQ*, initially published in 1995.[33] Goleman wasn't the first to investigate emotional intelligence, but he succeeded in popularizing the concept.

Goleman's book paved the way for a resurgence in the study and practice of emotional intelligence, sometimes called *emotional quotient* (EQ). EQ's main ideas have become a core concept in almost all models of human interaction. His five elements of EQ are self-regulation, self-awareness, motivation, empathy, and social skills.

As mentioned, there are other emotional intelligence models. We recommend looking at *The Handbook of Emotional Intelligence*, edited by Reuven Bar-On and James D. A. Parker.[34] There are a dozen or more research-oriented publications and websites where you can read more. Most EQ models are legitimate points of reference and will help guide you through conversations when you're working to demonstrate the best behaviors possible.

---

[33] Goleman, Daniel. Emotional Intelligence: 25th Anniversary Edition. Bloomsbury Publishing, 2020.

[34] Bar-On, Reuven, and James D. A. Parker. The Handbook of Emotional Intelligence: The Theory and Practice of Development, Evaluation, Education, and Application--at Home, School, and Workplace. Jossey-Bass, 2000.

Emotional intelligence skills framework

Based on our experiences during our combined 90 years of career adventures and the many organizations we've worked for, we'll summarize EQ into its core mandates.

1) Understand your impact on others.
2) Keep control of yourself in all situations.
3) Hesitate before speaking.
4) Prioritize the needs of others over your own needs.
5) Support and sustain the motivation of others.
6) Be positive and genuine.[35]

Mastering these six elements of your EQ takes a lifetime of dedicated work. After all, like Rome, you were not built in a day. However, all the behaviors suggested by these elements should be part of your long-term strategy to advocate more effectively for your loved ones in long-term care facilities.

This is a small window into our psyches: We have no trouble jumping into conversations, even if they're filled with emotional drama, even conflict. This is not always the best habit, and we've been working on developing the capability to *hesitate before speaking*. To a large degree, we've made progress via the *University of Hard Knocks*, a saying people from our generation will recognize immediately.

Emotional intelligence in practice

Every interaction is an opportunity to practice your emotional intelligence skills. As an advocate, you'll meet managers, caregivers, and staff members who facilitate or provide direct care. It may be helpful to think of emotional intelligence as a process rather than a moment.

When you meet someone who provides excellent care for your loved one or a manager of those people, acknowledge it. Everyone loves praise and gratitude beyond the friendly handshake and nod. When

---

[35] Smith, A. (2023). *No Time to Waste: Microbehaviors: Leveraging the Little Things to Become a Better Leader*. iUniverse.

you advocate for your loved one, we suggest you use this simple mental and verbal process:

Step 1—Accept the person for who they are. Avoid judgments about gender, race, ethnicity, national origin, culture, language, religion, disability, etc. Accept visible attributes like dress, hair, weight, height, jewelry, and other forms of personal adornment.

Step 2—Ask the person respectful and thoughtful questions. Then, listen to the answers. Later, we'll discuss the benefits of using curiosity as your superpower. Recall Stephen R. Covey's advice—*we should seek first to understand...*

Step 3—Express concern while talking about difficult situations the person faces. This may include admitting the issue with your loved one, which could be stressful. To complete Covey's quote—*and then [seek] to be understood.* [36]

Step 4—Conclude by showing sincere appreciation to the caregiver for helping your loved one.

Lack of emotional intelligence in others

You'll meet people in the long-term care environment who may have a distinct lack of emotional intelligence. They may not be trying to improve, either. We have known people across our long careers whose EQ did not consist of much more than *please* and *thank you*. It's a good start, but hopefully not the destination!

Champions should be mentally prepared to encounter people who fall into this category. They might lack emotional intelligence for many different reasons, including past trauma or a lack of good examples to emulate. And many other reasons, too.

Notwithstanding our suggestions in this chapter, the best thing to do may be to *take a break*—literally, step away. A person with little or no emotional intelligence will rarely respond well to receiving feedback

---

[36] Covey, Stephen R. *The 7 Habits of Highly Effective People: Powerful Lessons in Personal Change.* Simon and Schuster, 2013.

about the EQ void in their psyche. It's also true that few people like to be lectured on what they should do differently. We like the strategy captured in the idiomatic expression—*all roads lead to Rome*. Meaning: there are many different ways to achieve success.[37] We suggest finding someone who can better meet your needs and those of your loved ones.

When emotional intelligence includes a display of emotion

Champions should not fulfill their duties *devoid of emotion*. We hope we've not given you that impression. In the section below, plus the scenario, we offer thoughts on improving your emotional intelligence and putting those skills into practice. Let's be honest: we're emotional creatures and should expect strong sentiments to be present and verbalized.

One way to signal your emotions *and* avoid assigning blame is to begin commentaries with the phrase *I'm worried.* For example, *I'm worried we're missing a step in the care plan.* This sits much better than saying *I think you've missed a step in the care plan*. Or worse, *why can't you ever follow the steps in the care plan?* The first approach makes it a joint problem that can be solved together. The second and third approaches come laden with judgment.

The phrase *I'm worried* can also be delivered with passion. We'd counsel against a champion making observations to a caregiver or community staff member when they're uncontrollably angry. *Walk it off first.* But frustration, anxiety, sadness, and disappointment are all fair game in a conversation, provided they reflect what's in your mind.[38]

---

[37] Osmond, C. (2023, June 24). *All Roads Lead to Rome - Origin & Meaning.* GRAMMARIST. https://grammarist.com/proverb/all-roads-lead-to-rome/
[38] King, S. (2013). *Brag, Worry, Wonder, Bet: A Manager's Guide to Giving Feedback.* iUniverse.

Improving your emotional intelligence skills

- **Conduct research**—Read books about emotional intelligence like Daniel Goleman's *Emotional Intelligence*, Mark T. Coleman's *Emotional Intelligence 2.0*, and Jeanne Segal's *The Language of Emotional Intelligence.*
- **Practice mindfulness**—Stay focused on the present and think before you speak.
- **Promote collaboration**—See the people who care for your loved one as teammates. Use words like *we* and *our* and give them the benefit of the doubt during tough times.
- **Expand vocabulary**—Get better at explaining your feelings without confrontation by learning new words and phrases.
- **Seek advice**—Ask others how they would handle a challenging situation and bounce ideas off them.

Scenario—emotional intelligence skills

It's 10:00 a.m., and you discover that your father has not been toileted, dressed, or fed upon arriving in his memory care community.

One Way	A Better Way
Champion: Dad is still in bed and smells like he needs to be changed. Has he even been served breakfast today? **Administrator:** I'm sorry, who is your father? What room is he in? **Champion:** How can you not know my father? He's been here for six months! What's going on here anyway? **Administrator:** I'm sorry, I don't know your father; we've over 50 residents here, but if you tell me his name and room number, I will check in with the staff. **Champion:** That's not good enough. Dad needs help right now. He shouldn't have to wait for the basics of getting dressed and fed. It's after 10:00 a.m. already. Who's responsible for this failure? **Administrator:** I understand you're upset, but I still need to know who your father is and what room he's in.	**Champion:** Hello! My name is Edward Miller, and I am the son of Henry Miller in Room 207. **Administrator:** Yes, Mr. Miller, how can I help you? **Champion:** I was just in to see Dad and it looks like he hasn't been out of bed yet this morning, and I am betting he needs to be changed. Can you help me sort this out? **Administrator:** I see. I haven't heard of anything about your father, but I can look into it. **Champion:** That would be great if you could check with your staff. Is there someone else I can ask? I just barged in on you unannounced. **Administrator:** That's a great idea. Let's find one of the aides who has been on duty today and see what we can find out. **Champion:** Let's do it.

From experience with administrators and staff, we know the approach in the column on the right above will create much more positive action than on the left. There may be an accountable party on staff in the community who should have awakened, changed, dressed, and fed your loved one, but seeking to find someone to blame in the moment rarely achieves the desired outcome. There will be time later for a follow-up and setting of expectations.

If you can see yourself responding as the champion did, as shown on the right— congratulations!—you're showing a lot of emotional intelligence. But you have more work to do if you see yourself responding more like the dialog on the left. In our experience, we rarely see one approach fully or the other. Frequently, champions fall somewhere in between, neither fully exhibiting emotional intelligence nor entirely discarding it.

Recall St. Francis de Sales' famous words:

You catch more flies with a spoonful of honey than a barrel of vinegar. [39]

---

[39] Oblates of St. Francis de Sales. "St. Francis de Sales — Oblates of St. Francis de Sales," n.d. https://www.oblates.org/st-francis-wisdom.

NOTES

Chapter 10—Understanding Your Loved One's Rights

Don't Tread on Me

Don't Tread on Me is a motto attached to the 1775 Gadsden flag, the design of which is credited to Christopher Gadsden, a Continental Army Brigadier General. The flag was used by the Continental Marines until the Stars and Stripes were adopted as the flag for the United States. The flag boasts the defiant message below a coiled rattlesnake on a yellow background. You've probably seen it here and there.

The motto conveys vigilance and readiness to defend. The American Colonies wanted their rights and freedoms protected. We think this mindset is appropriate for advocates safeguarding the rights of loved ones in structured community settings.[40] [41] When you become a champion, you must also become acquainted with the fundamental principles governing their rights.

Basic resident rights

A person living in a long-term care community maintains the same freedoms, privileges, and rights as any citizen of the United States or someone residing here. However, due to the artificial environment of long-term care, your vigilance level as a champion must be higher overall. This is especially true for memory care residents who are in cognitive decline and aren't able to defend themselves. Regular visits to the community, with your mental checklist at the ready, will help to ensure your loved one is being treated appropriately. Finally, each community should provide written leases and resident handbooks

---

[40] Bickerton, James. "Gadsden Flag Meaning Explained and Its Revolutionary Origins." *Newsweek*, August 31, 2023. https://www.newsweek.com/gadsden-flag-meaning-explained-1823467.

[41] Seo, Krish. "Don't Tread on Me Flag - Origins and Significance." *American Flags* (blog), January 23, 2024. https://www.americanflags.com/blog/post/dont-tread-on-me-flag-origins-significance.

governing resident-tenant rights. We have been told about community administrators enforcing *unwritten* guidelines, leading to champions and loved ones requesting to *show me [where it's written]*.

20 essential resident rights

Below is our distillation of the 20 essential rights of your loved one in a long-term care community. This is not an exhaustive list. Each numbered item can be expounded upon.[42]

i.	To freely exercise rights as a citizen.
ii.	To be free from retaliation after exercising rights provided by law or rule.
iii.	To be treated with dignity and respect.
iv.	To have the opportunity to understand services and select or refuse.
v.	To participate in care plan creation and any revisions or updates.
vi.	To receive information about the assessment of needed services and fees.
vii.	To be free from neglect and verbal, mental, physical, or sexual abuse.
viii.	To receive services that protect privacy and dignity.
ix.	To have prompt access to records and receive copies.
x.	To keep medical and other records confidential.
xi.	To associate and communicate privately with any person.
xii.	To send and receive emails unopened and have access to a private phone.
xiii.	To be free from physical restraints and inappropriate psychoactive medications.
xiv.	To manage personal financial affairs.
xv.	To participate in social activities.
xvi.	To be free of any agreement that waives protected rights or community liability.
xvii.	To voice grievances and suggest changes without retaliation.
xviii.	To have a safe, secure, and homelike environment.

---

[42] Excellent online resources discuss resident rights. For more detailed information and resources, please see the End Notes and Tools section, *Resident Rights.*

xix.   To be free of discrimination on any basis.

xx.   To receive information if requested to move out of the community.[43] [44]

Questions for loved ones about their community experiences

We discussed earlier the need to make curiosity your superpower. Using this skill for a constant dialog stream is critical to maintaining a loved one's rights. For loved ones in assisted living, this is a straightforward process. Most of the residents we know are eager to engage in social interactions with family members and friends *from the outside.* In our experience, a few well-considered questions to your loved one do the trick.

- Who are the residents you like the most? Do you enjoy visiting with them? Why?
- Who are the caregivers you like the most? Are there any you don't like? Why?
- How was <insert meal> today? What did you eat? Were the servers polite?
- What activities have you attended recently? Did you enjoy them? Why?
- How did your appointment with <insert healthcare provider> go? Were your questions answered? How comfortable are you with the care you're receiving?
- Your bath was scheduled for yesterday; how did it go? Do you have any concerns?
- Is your laundry done on time and put away to your liking?
- When you use your call button, does someone come quickly? How long do you wait?
- Are you getting your medication on time? Have there been significant delays or incorrect medication?

---

43 "National Consumer Voice," n.d. https://ltcombudsman.org/issues/residents-rights.
44 LII / Legal Information Institute. "42 CFR § 483.10 - Resident Rights.," n.d. https://www.law.cornell.edu/cfr/text/42/483.10.

Discussing a loved one in memory care could sound very different. You probably won't quiz them with questions, for instance. Instead, you'll need to rely more on discussions with caregivers.

- How was <insert name> appetite at <insert meal>? Are they eating enough?
- How did it go when you got <insert name> up this morning? Do you have any concerns?
- Did <insert name> receive their new medication today? Are you noticing any problems?
- Is <insert name> joining in on activities? Which ones do they enjoy the most?
- Were there any issues when you gave <insert name> a bath yesterday?
- Are there supplies <insert name> needs? Is anything running low?

There may be a need in the memory care environment to *shop for answers.* This means asking the same question of different caregivers on various shifts—weekday, weekend, day, and night. We recently encountered a situation where a caregiver on the day shift had zero knowledge about the nighttime or morning routines. Likewise, a nighttime caregiver could not answer questions about mealtimes. This also applies to administering medications, which could occur on any shift.

Vigilant observation is your friend in memory care settings. We constantly check the following since it gives us a flavor of how things are going.

- Are the garbage cans emptied? Do they have plastic liners?
- How full is the laundry basket? Are clothes stowed in dressers and closets properly?
- Is your loved one wearing clean clothes? Is their dignity being preserved?
- Is your loved one frequently in need of changing when you visit?
- How does your loved one react when caregivers enter the room?
- Is the cafeteria cleaned up between meals? Are there dirty dishes on the dining tables?

- Are beverages and snacks available to your loved one between meals? How?
- How respectful and *in the moment* are caregivers when you pose questions?

Frequent areas of complaint for long-term care communities

Turning our attention to the most frequent complaints state and other oversight agencies received, we can see some concerns are specific to fundamental resident rights. In 2019, the National Opinion Research Center (NORC) at the University of Chicago published a brief titled *Protecting Rights and Preventing Abuse: Handling Resident Complaints in Long-Term Care Facilities.*

We're quoting directly from the brief that NORC published with the top ten areas of complaint. These complaint areas are relatively steady from one year to the next.

1. **Discharge/eviction**—planning, notice, procedure, implementation, and abandonment.
2. **Medication**—administration, organization.
3. **Foodservice**—quantity, quality, variation, choice, condiments, utensils, menu.
4. **Dignity**—staff attitudes.
5. **Equipment/building**—disrepair, hazard, poor lighting, fire safety, not secure.
6. **Cleanliness**—pests, general housekeeping.
7. **Resident conflict**—roommates.
8. **Accident**—injuries of unknown origin, falls, improper handling.
9. **Personal property**—lost, stolen, used by others, destroyed, withheld from a resident.
10. **Care plans/resident assessments**—inadequate, failure to follow plan or physician orders.[45]

---

[45] Nguyen, Kim, Ph.D., Sarah Downey MPP, and Emily White MA. *Protecting Rights and Preventing Abuse: Handling Resident Complaints in Long-Term Care Facilities.* eBook. National Opinion Research Center at the University of Chicago, 2019. https://acl.gov/sites/default/files/programs/2020-10/NORC%20Research%20Brief_Handling%20Resident%20Complaints_508.pdf.

Early identification and discussion of any concerns is the best approach. Common sense only sometimes wins when it comes to caregiving. While this is disappointing, champions must rely on more than logic.

A recent situation highlighted this for us. A loved one was discovered several times to have two incontinence briefs on at the same time. Typically, there would be one brief with a single incontinence pad. When the question was posed about why two briefs were being put on the loved one, the answer was the second brief could be pulled up immediately after removing the soiled brief. Is that efficient? Maybe. Except two briefs create a situation where a loved one might remain in a soiled brief longer, promoting skin irritation and infection. And where does it end? With three or four briefs stacked, one on top of the other. We fear no common sense was applied.

Submitting a complaint about a long-term care community

Only some problems in a long-term care community rise to the level of a formal complaint to a government watchdog group, like a state's Long-Term Care Ombudsmen Program. But, if a complaint becomes necessary, it's essential to provide specific details such as the names of affected individuals and staff, dates, times, and a short description of the incident. Facilities must inform residents of their complaint procedures and prominently display contact information for relevant agencies. Filing a complaint does not mean the problem will be automatically or quickly remedied.

Upon receiving a complaint, regulatory agencies acknowledge receipt within a specific timeframe and may conduct onsite investigations if warranted. Investigations follow state and federal guidelines, with findings documented and shared with the complainant. Communities found in violation may be required to submit a plan of correction, and enforcement actions could range from citations to fines or license revocation, depending on the severity of the non-compliance.

Filing formal complaints is sometimes necessary to address severe issues within long-term care communities. Understanding the process and available resources empowers residents and advocates to uphold the rights and well-being of individuals in these settings. Vigilance and advocacy are essential in ensuring accountability and promoting quality care for all residents.

NOTES

Chapter 11—Performing the Role of Agent

Champions may or may not serve as the legal representative or guardian of an adult family member or friend in a long-term care community. We'll use the word *agent* in this chapter to identify these special accountabilities.

The decision about whether an advocate plays the add-on responsibility of an agent is usually the result of an extensive conversation with the loved one and family members. Appointment to the role of agent is a legal process involving specific documents whose requirements to be valid vary from state to state.

We want to reiterate we're not attorneys. Nothing in *Champions Needed* constitutes legal advice. You should always consult your attorney for advice and counsel. Representation and decision-making authority are frequently complex and involve many variables, requiring specialized expertise.

If you need a place to start researching legal matters about your senior loved one, we suggest visiting the American Association of Retired Persons website, Legal Counsel for the Elderly. This AARP service is free and covers the gamut of issues from powers-of-attorney to elder abuse claims. Here's the address of that website: https://www.aarp.org/legal-counsel-for-elderly/.[46]

Through the rest of this chapter, we'll discuss *the basics*—enough for you to get a taste of what being an agent means and some of the most urgent issues to address.

---

[46] "Protecting, Empowering & Advocating for DC Older Adults," n.d. https://www.aarp.org/legal-counsel-for-elderly/.

Three types of legal agents

An agent is authorized by another individual, the principal (commonly the loved one), to act on their behalf in legal matters or transactions. This authorization grants the agent the power to make decisions, enter into contracts, and perform other legal acts as if they were the principal themselves. Such capabilities are typically granted via a formally executed document like a *power-of-attorney*. Agents come in three standard configurations:

- **General agent**—A general agent possesses broad authority but is limited to specific transactions, such as contracts, real estate, business relationships, medical, etc.
- **Special agent**—A special agent possesses more limited authority and is sometimes appointed for one-time transactions, e.g., purchase/sale of real property.
- **Universal agent**—A universal agent can speak for the principal in all ways and possess comprehensive authority over a wide range of potential transactions, including those stated under the general agent definition.[47]

The relationship between the agent and the principal is governed by Agency Law, which dictates both parties' duties, rights, and liabilities. Key elements of such an arrangement include the agent's obligation to act loyally and in the principal's best interest. An adjoining principle is decisions are legally binding when the agent acts within their authority.[48]

In situations where a loved one has been declared incapacitated, and *there is legal documentation* supporting the appointment of an agent, the transition of decision-making to the agent is generally straightforward. The appointed agent can make important decisions about finances and, if specified, healthcare.

---

[47] You can consult many online resources about different types of agents and other legal terminology, including www.lawdistrict.com, www.law.cornell.edu, and www.dictionary.law.com.

[48] See LII/Legal Information Institute under "Agency," n.d. https://www.law.cornell.edu/wex/agency.

In situations where a loved one is declared incapacitated, and *there is no legal documentation* supporting the appointment of an agent, the transition of decision-making is frequently not easy nor straightforward. While many legal jurisdictions will favor appointing a spouse as an agent, this is not a certainty and may require court filings and appearances. It's also possible family members, other than the spouse, may feel they're better suited to be the loved one's agent.

An *agent* and an *advocate* are not necessarily the same person. An agent could simultaneously perform the role of an advocate and vice versa. A frequent variation on this arrangement is that one agent handles all financial and legal matters while a different agent is appointed to make healthcare decisions.

We don't have a recommendation on which path to follow when appointing an agent. Individual circumstances should dictate the outcome. We're familiar with numerous situations where duties are split across family members. We also know of other cases where the responsibilities are concentrated on one person only.

Communication is required in all cases among family members and third parties such as the long-term care community, physicians and other providers, investment and banking organizations, insurance companies, etc.

Power of Attorney triggering events

In our experience, *when* an agent begins to exercise authority for their loved one, it always creates a debate within the family. In circumstances where a capable and willing spouse is involved, the decision about *agent activation* is more straightforward to resolve. However, when the spouse is no longer alive or able to fill the agent role, the question about who the agent is and when their authority begins can be fractious and difficult. Governing documents should be very clear on this point.

Time is not your friend here. There is always less time than you think. We can conclusively state that waiting until the last minute to implement legally binding solutions is an excellent way to put strain on your loved one, family members, and friends.

You could be an advocate or champion without absolute authority to make healthcare decisions for your loved one. Unfortunately, this is not uncommon, and it may cause you to metaphorically *look over your shoulder*, wondering if the designated agent will swoop in and make countervailing recommendations or decisions.

We know of multiple cases where instructions and appropriate legal documents were implemented many years before the need arose. This is the best of many possible ways to approach the challenge. In one case, the 2nd oldest child of an aging parent received an appointment as a universal agent *immediately* upon execution of the POA versus waiting for an incapacitating event. In another case, the oldest child of an aging parent received an appointment as a universal agent *only if the parent could not make their own decisions.*

Here are a few POA triggering events for you to consider as an agent/advocate:

- **Unavailability and temporary impairment**—triggering event is the principal's inability to communicate healthcare decisions for themselves due to being unconscious, undergoing a surgical procedure, in a medically-induced coma, or the result of a physician's evaluation. Keyword: *temporary.*
- **Specific medical conditions**—triggering event is the principal being diagnosed with certain medical conditions such as a terminal illness or severe cognitive impairment, including advancing dementia or Alzheimer's disease.
- **Total incapacitation**—triggering event is the principal being declared unable to manage their affairs or make decisions for themselves due to enduring physical, mental, or emotional impairment. The agreement of more than one medical professional is typically required to create such a determination, and sometimes, it involves the oversight of a court of law.

Special case of *Do Not Resuscitate* instructions

We've debated the value of discussing *Do Not Resuscitate (DNR)* orders in *Champions Needed.* Given the critical issues surrounding the authority given to agents, as outlined in the various legal documents we've examined, we feel it would be remiss to exclude DNR information. There is no more intimate, personal issue a champion can discuss with a loved one than circumstances under which life-saving treatments will or will not be rendered.

In simple terms, a DNR consists of a written order by a physician instructing healthcare providers to withhold Cardiopulmonary Resuscitation (CPR) if a patient's heart stops or they stop breathing. DNR instructions are most often issued in cases of severe illness or end-of-life situations and countermand performing chest compressions, inserting advanced airways, administering cardiac resuscitation drugs, providing ventilator assistance, or defibrillation.[49]

Most states now require more than the language shown in a POA or Advanced Medical Directive to withhold CPR in the moment of an emergency. Instead, regulations and policies necessitate completing a form, signed by an attending physician, and wearing a bracelet or other item of plainly visible jewelry to communicate DNR instructions. To understand the requirements of the state in which your loved one lives, we suggest searching online for *<insert name of state> DNR instructions.*

Advocates and their loved ones should be open and transparent about DNR instructions. Conversations with loved ones who fully possess their faculties are not easy. Imagining the moment of one's demise is the hardest thing humans can do. Whether religion, philosophy, or something else drives the creation of a DNR, it's usually an emotional conversation.

---

[49] Pope, Thaddeus Mason. "Confidentiality and HIPAA." Merck Manuals Consumer Version, December 6, 2023. https://www.merckmanuals.com/home/fundamentals/legal-and-ethical-issues/confidentiality-and-hipaa.

Ultimately, a champion follows their loved one's direction about end-of-life scenarios. We strongly encourage the conversation about DNRs to take place long before the need arises. And the embedding of specific instructions in the POA under which an agent/advocate operates.

NOTES

Chapter 12—Individual and Community Emergencies

Obvious but essential—you won't always be present

A healthcare emergency can strike your loved one without warning, and you'll likely not be physically present. Recognizing this limitation is monumentally important. Such awareness should prompt champions to prepare proactively for health emergencies.

We've seen residents of long-term care communities transported by ambulance due to several urgent issues. Falls are the most common and, as reported by the CDC, highlighted earlier, all too often end in tragedy. But other sudden ailments can just as easily overcome your loved one: a too-high blood pressure reading, sudden chest pains, dizziness, and shortness of breath. Moments like this can and do arrive frequently.

Long-term care communities are generally vigilant and have protocols to follow in a health emergency. The agent or advocate is immediately contacted. And if the first person on the contact list is unavailable, they'll move down the list. Despite best intentions, locating the advocate quickly is sometimes challenging. Time is of the essence for the resident. Ambulances will come and go, and your loved one could be in the hospital ER before you even know there's a problem.

In one emergency we know about, the agent-of-record was informed their loved one in memory care had been transported to the ER. The advocate jumped in the car to drive an hour to the supposed hospital. Just short of arrival, the champion received a call from the attending doctor, who provided a status update. The doctor casually mentioned the hospital's name as they said their goodbyes. To the advocate's surprise, their loved one had been taken to a different hospital entirely. Emergency compounded by human error. Was it the advocate's fault? The community's? Honestly, we don't know. Paperwork completed long ahead of time identified which hospital to use.

Please read this as a cautionary tale. Our point is that champions must be ready to handle any possible scenario with zero warning.

Essential documents

Our earlier chapter on organization and documentation listed items you should always have handy. When a loved one is in a health emergency, it's not the time for a champion to search for important information. We've reiterated the list of essential documents below.

- ID cards for Medicare, Medicaid, Advantage, and Supplemental insurance plans.
- List of medications taken with dosage amounts and times.
- Advance directives showing your loved one's agents and instructions.
- DNR documents, if any, and other State-required items (e.g., forms, bracelets, etc.).
- Contact emails and phone numbers for community management, physicians, nurses, and caregivers.

We encourage you to keep copies of these essentials in your car, phone, home and loved one's room. *Don't take anything for granted.*

Transporting to the hospital emergency room

One of the immediate questions posed in the advent of a healthcare emergency is whether transport to a hospital is required. There are no absolute standards governing the response to this question. Most communities have *policies* that inform the decision. For example, transporting after a fall is a standard policy requirement.

The American College of Emergency Physicians published guidelines for calling 9-1-1in an emergent health care situation.[50] Below are four explicit scenarios when you or the long-term care community should call for emergency transport:

---

[50] "When-and When Not-to Call an Ambulance," n.d.
https://www.emergencyphysicians.org/article/er101/when---and-when-not---to-call-an-ambulance.

- Chest pains, difficulty breathing, sudden confusion, or altered mental state.
- Choking and the need to perform the Heimlich maneuver, or similar, or back blows.
- The heart stops, and CPR is needed. *Call 9-1-1 first!*
- Moving the person may risk further injury.

Conventional wisdom suggests calling 9-1-1 *when in doubt*. We agree, but 9-1-1 is not the best answer in all cases. Sometimes, an ambulance should be obtained using a private transport service or even a wheelchair van. The decision depends on the severity of the health emergency. If any of the four situations above are part of the scenario, quickly call 9-1-1.

As a thoughtful and cost-conscious advocate, you may consider transporting your loved one in a private vehicle instead of an ambulance. We hope you'll consider this carefully before doing so. If your loved one usually uses a wheelchair, this may not be a good idea. If they use a walker and rarely a wheelchair, it's probably a safer bet. However, many experts warn of transfer-related injuries. We encourage you to consult a healthcare professional in advance.

You should discuss protocols for emergency transportation with community management as soon as your loved one moves in. Emergencies don't arrive on a schedule convenient to you or your loved ones. Knowing the expectations will go a long way to ensuring a calm and confident demeanor if/when a situation arises.

If you decide *against* the community's recommendation to transport your loved one to the emergency room, you'll be asked to sign a document confirming your decision. The document will be full of legalese. You shouldn't be concerned about signing if you're confident in your decision. If you have any doubts, the document will prompt you to reconsider.

Community emergencies

Unfortunately, champions will face more than healthcare emergencies. Some common hazards a community should plan for include severe weather (wind, rain, snow), natural disasters (earthquakes, hurricanes, tornadoes, floods, wildfires), in-community fires, equipment failure (plumbing, electrical, HVAC), power outages, and active shooter scenarios. We've personally experienced several of these situations.

Take, for example, a power outage. We know of a night-time situation when the local municipal power company, including the assisted living and memory care community, inadvertently cut the power to half the city. Upon investigation, there was no estimate of when power would be restored. Nothing operated in the community except battery-powered emergency lighting in the hallways, and all residents were instructed to stay in the lit areas.

When the power went out, one advocate we know rushed to the community to find their loved one reclined in an electric lift lounger. The loved one had no way to get up since the chair couldn't be restored to a sitting position. How long would they need to stay reclined in the lounger? Nobody knew. The quick-thinking advocate rallied four healthcare aides to lift the loved one out of the lounger and into a wheelchair.

There should be a community policy or protocol to rely upon when the power goes out. The routine problem of power outages, which is *always* inconvenient, can rapidly become a massive issue for residents. Advocates must be prepared to step in and ensure that loved ones are adequately cared for when such things happen.

Community responsibilities

According to state and federal regulations, long-term care communities must create an emergency preparedness program. Programs must include these and other components:

1) An emergency plan is informed via a building-by-building risk assessment, resident population evaluation, continuity of operations, and a process for collaboration with local, tribal, state, or federal emergency preparedness officials.
2) The development of policies and procedures based on the emergency plan, which is updated at least annually.
3) A communications, training, testing, and notifications plan for staff, third-party providers, physicians, etc.[51]

Skilled nursing facilities must meet additional requirements, including emergency generator placement and maintenance.

Advocates should proactively review the emergency preparedness program with community management. You can request copies of policies and procedures. We especially encourage you to understand what the emergency plan calls for when evacuation of residents is required. As stated earlier in this chapter, *you probably won't be present during an emergency.*

Another cautionary tale: we know of a community emergency where the kitchen in the community caught fire after the evening meal service was concluded. Per plan, residents were evacuated from the building's interior to the exterior using all available exits. Residents in wheelchairs were moved to safe locations while the Fire Department extinguished the flames. The weather was cold and rainy, so residents had blankets wrapped around their shoulders when wheeled out. So far, so good.

---

[51] LII / Legal Information Institute. "42 CFR § 483.73 - Emergency Preparedness.," n.d. https://www.law.cornell.edu/cfr/text/42/483.73#:~:text=%C2%A7%20483.7 3%20Emergency%20preparedness.,the%20requirements%20of%20this%20s ection.

After the fire was out and the local all-clear sign was given to return inside, several residents were left outside, forgotten, in the inclement weather. Almost two hours passed before caregivers performed a bed check and discovered these residents were missing. Advocates and family members were informed that there had been an emergency the next day, but not that their loved ones had been left out in the cold.

What can we learn from this situation? And what could champions do in the aftermath? Here are some possibilities:

- Request updating and clarifying communication protocols. Being informed late is unacceptable and increases anxiety and distrust.
- Request reliable accountability systems for emergencies.
- Request clarity on steps to be taken after an emergency, including re-entry procedures and an immediate bed check to ensure all residents are accounted for.
- Request regular training and drills for staff, ensuring emergency procedures are effective, and roles are clear.
- Request adequate supplies, incl. warm blankets, clothing, etc.
- Request care assessments for residents negatively impacted.
- Request post-emergency debriefings to discuss what went well and what did not, leading to possible improvements.

Advocates must constantly ensure that loved ones' rights, whether present during an emergency, are maintained. We've alluded to the fact that we're not bashful when speaking up in situations requiring attention from the communities where our loved ones live. You shouldn't be, either.

American humorist Josh Billings said:

I hate to be a kicker [complainer]...I always long for peace, But the wheel that does the squeaking Is the one that gets the grease.[52]

---

[52] "Dictionary.com | Meanings & Definitions of English Words." In *Dictionary.Com*, n.d. https://www.dictionary.com/browse/squeaky-wheel-gets-the-grease.

NOTES

Chapter 13—Managing Family Relationships

Family relationships–in context

Families are often regarded as the cornerstone of our lives. Most comprise an intricate matrix of relationships woven with emotions, shared histories, and, perhaps most significantly, attitudes. The attitudes held within the familial realm are pivotal in shaping the dynamics, fostering harmony or discord. Attitudes serve as the architects of our interpersonal landscapes. These profoundly ingrained predispositions, formed by cultural influences, personal experiences, and societal norms, mold how family members perceive one another and the world around them.

Similar to how a pebble creates ripples reaching far beyond its initial point of impact in a pond, behaviors springing from long-established attitudes generate ripples and sometimes waves. Positive behaviors like empathy, respect, and open-mindedness pave the way for healthy communication and understanding. Conversely, negative behaviors, like judgment, resentment, or stubbornness, can cast a shadow, darkening the family dynamic and leaving lasting scars.

The overarching objective for family management by advocates is to create a space where positive behaviors thrive and foster open dialogue, allowing family members to express their thoughts and emotions. Family dynamics may be the most challenging component of your role as a champion.

We know of many situations where well-meaning, non-advocate relatives of loved ones in long-term care are capable of putting a foot firmly in their mouths. For example, the sibling of an advocate said in front of their loved one in an LTC community that they would *rather die alone in their home than move to assisted living.* Once the words escaped the sibling's lips, there was no recalling them. The loved one was upset, and the advocate was left to smooth out the situation. So much for a positive family dynamic!

Family relationships—ever-flexible

The ability of family members to adapt and adjust their behaviors is crucial for the healthy maintenance of family bonds. A rigid attitude can impede growth and create tension. A flexible and adaptive mindset allows for the ebb and flow of relationships, nurturing a sense of unity despite the inevitable challenges that arise. Advocates are often called upon to exhibit high degrees of flexibility when everyone else seems to have turned to stone.

The beneficiaries of functioning, healthy relationships are the loved ones who are obliged to rely entirely on their family for support. Can you imagine how disturbing it might be for a loved one to witness an argument among their children about which medical treatment might be best for them? Holding a reasonable and respectful conversation is always a good option. But a loud difference of opinion creates confusion, doubt, and anxiety.

In our experience, most family members want to be involved in decisions about their loved one's well-being. However, challenges may arise when needs evolve, requiring difficult choices and transitions that impact family relationships. Advocates lead by example. A champion can foster an environment of kindness and cooperation through compassion and understanding. When advocates exhibit unilateral decision-making behaviors, frustration grows, and trust is lost.

In one of our families, the widow of a close family member was unaccountably absent from their home and did not answer her phone. A sister of the deceased family member went repeatedly to the empty house, trying to understand what happened. During one visit, the sister stumbled on the house's new owners, who were in the process of moving in!

Upon inquiry, the sibling discovered the widow's brother, who was the designated POA and *theoretical* advocate, had sold the house, had the widow declared incapacitated, and moved her into a long-term care community. The widow's five step-children knew nothing of this chain of events. Nor did the six siblings of the deceased family member. It happened very fast, in under a month. Many unhappy discussions ensued, but the damage was done.

Family relationships–conflict is inevitable

Family conflicts and disagreements are inevitable. However, the way champions address them can significantly impact the outcome. Provoking or fueling confrontation often escalates tensions and impedes constructive dialogue, making it challenging to reach beneficial resolutions. Advocates should approach conflicts calmly and with a level head, seeking to understand all parties' underlying concerns and perspectives. This is good advice when dealing with family, friends, or caregivers.

Constructive solutions lie in active listening and intentional empathy. Advocates, with some thought, can cleverly de-escalate volatile situations and promote collaborative problem-solving. This can be achieved by refraining from aggressive language, exhibiting emotional maturity, and maintaining self-control. Conflict generates abundant energy champions can channel into finding common ground and working towards solutions centered on their loved one's needs.

When we assume the responsibility of advocating for our loved ones in a senior living community setting, it's natural to expect support and involvement from other family members. However, take this with a grain of salt. Be realistic about what each individual can contribute based on their circumstances, availability, and relationship dynamics. Some people will have different capacities or willingness to participate in caregiving responsibilities.

Some family members may have competing priorities, such as work or caring for other family members. Placing expectations on family members will only increase your pressure if they cannot fulfill their commitments. Develop foresight for each person's strengths and limitations so you can collaborate more effectively and allocate responsibilities accordingly.

Conflict management styles

The need for conflict management among family members involves acknowledging differing opinions and finding compromises to ensure the best outcomes. Understanding your conflict management style can significantly aid in building and maintaining productive relationships with your loved ones, family members, and others.

A helpful tool for assessing conflict management styles is the Thomas-Kilmann Conflict Mode Instrument (TKI), developed by Dr. Kenneth W. Thomas and Dr. Ralph H. Kilmann in 1977.[53] The TKI has become a widely used tool for understanding how individuals respond to conflict. It helps people grasp how different conflict management styles impact interpersonal dynamics, empowering them to choose the most suitable approach. The TKI identifies five styles: [54]

1) **Accommodating**—Unassertive and cooperative, accommodating prioritizes the concerns of others over one's own, often leading to self-sacrifice.
2) **Avoiding**—Unassertive and uncooperative, avoiding sidesteps conflicts altogether, either by postponing them or diplomatically avoiding confrontation.
3) **Collaborating**—Assertive and cooperative, collaborating seeks to find mutually beneficial solutions by addressing all concerns.
4) **Competing**—This style is assertive and uncooperative, focusing on winning at the expense of others.

---

[53] Kilmann. "An Overview of the TKI Assessment Tool." Kilmann Diagnostics, January 8, 2022. https://kilmanndiagnostics.com/brief-overview-of-the-tki-assessment/#:~:text=Kilmann%2C%20co%2Dauthor%20of%20the,underlying%20dimensions%3A%20assertiveness%20and%20cooperativeness.

[54] ____. "Take the Thomas-Kilmann Conflict Mode Instrument (TKI). Take This Assessment Tool and Discover Which of the Five Conflict Modes You Might Be Using Too Much or Too Little... or Just Right." Kilmann Diagnostics, December 24, 2020. https://kilmanndiagnostics.com/overview-thomas-kilmann-conflict-mode-instrument-tki/.

5) **Compromising**—Intermediate between assertiveness and cooperativeness, compromising aims to find practical solutions partially satisfying both parties.

No one conflict style is perfect

Each of the TKI styles has advantages and potential pitfalls. For example, while accommodating can create a sense of goodwill and trust, overusing it may result in your ideas and concerns needing to be noticed. On the other hand, competing can be effective in urgent situations or when advocating for critical issues. Still, it may lead to strained relationships if overused.

Reflecting on your conflict management style and considering how it aligns with different situations can help you resolve conflicts more effectively and maintain peace. We're a mix of all styles but generally approach the world and its conflict with a primary and secondary type. The TKI suggests *collaborating* as a hoped-for default position when disputes arise.

Understanding the five different conflict styles will help you in your champion role. If you want to go deeper, you should take the TKI assessment alone or with other family members. There are various online locations where you can complete the evaluation.[55]

Be prepared to forgive and reconcile

Over the years, as champions, we've learned that managing conflict requires *forgiveness* and *reconciliation*. Differentiating between the two concepts is essential. Understanding the various dimensions of forgiveness and reconciliation will benefit all involved and promote healing.

Forgiveness frequently paves the way for reconciliation. It's a multidimensional and deliberate choice encompassing intrapersonal

---

[55] Here are two alternatives for taking the Thomas-Kilmann Conflict Mode Instrument— https://kilmanndiagnostics.com/assessments/thomas-kilmann-instrument-one-assessment-person/, OR https://careerassessmentsite.com/tests/thomas-kilmann-tki-tests/about-the-thomas-kilmann-conflict-mode-instrument-tki/.

                 © WatchWorks Management Consulting LLC

and interpersonal facets. Forgiveness involves relinquishing self-justified feelings of *being right* and recognizing the shared humanity between the forgiver and supposed offender. It can release the burden of past hurts and reclaim agency over your life. Studies have shown that forgiveness contributes to better health outcomes, stronger relationships, and reduced anxiety, improving individual and group well-being.

Reconciliation, on the other hand, entails a *restoration* of a previously functional relationship and the cultivation of peace. It starts with acknowledging past grievances, building new, positive experiences, and facilitating broader change. Reconciliation plays a monumental role—helping rebuild and sustain family peace, bridging divides, and promoting cohesion.[56]

Since we're not experts on forgiveness or reconciliation, we recommend Hollis Green's book *Power of Forgiveness and Reconciliation: Forgiveness is the Sunrise of Reconciliation* (Greenwine Family Books, March 2020).

Significant others of champions

Advocates with significant others probably regularly find themselves between the proverbial rock and a hard place. You may be spending much of your available time tending to the healthcare of a loved one in long-term care to the detriment of the relationship with your life mate. It's easy for this to happen since the urgent matters of the loved one for whom you are the chosen champion tend to overwhelm all other considerations and commitments.

There's no easy way for us to say this, so we'll tell the hard truth: Ignoring the needs of your life mate is akin to juggling firesticks doused with gasoline. If you persist in this behavior, you will end up in flames. It's not a pretty picture!

---

[56] "Chapter 28. Spirituality and Community Building | Section 4. Forgiveness and Reconciliation | Main Section | Community ToolBox." n.d. https://ctb.ku.edu/en/table-of-contents/spirituality-and-community-building/forgiveness-and-reconciliation/main.

We discussed earlier the inevitability of emergencies for your loved one in assisted living or memory care. Please understand what we're saying. If there is an emergency, you must deal with it or find a reasonable substitute. Some things *can't wait.* Yet, to put a fine point on it, some things *can wait.* If you have a dinner date with your significant other, you should do your best to keep it. If your grandchild is celebrating a birthday, you should be there. If you need a break from the advocate routine, you should take it.

Prioritizing the needs of others in your family is not a treasonous act. Loved ones in long-term care are counting on you. But by definition, you aren't present 7x24x365. We advise you as much as possible to stick to a schedule known to you, your significant other, and your loved one. Your loved ones intuitively know you have a life outside their long-term care community. The problem is they have only a limited ability to participate in it. Recognize that they are mourning the loss of their freedom and your companionship, so occasionally, you may experience *transference* where you suddenly shoulder blame and guilt.

For loved ones in memory care, the challenge is more significant because your level of vigilance must be higher. Predictability, we have some advice for you here, too! Relationships with caregivers of your loved ones in memory care are paramount. They are your eyes and ears when you are not present. Keeping a tight schedule for memory care visits is probably unnecessary, mainly if your loved one can no longer track times and dates. Your presence comforts loved ones in memory whenever you can be there. But, again, ensure you are also meeting the needs of your significant other.

Tips for managing family relationships

Recognizing there is no foolproof way to maintain positive family relationships and avoid conflicts, we offer up a few tips that have worked for us:

- **Communicate regularly**—Use all available technology to stay in touch with family members, provide updates on your loved one's condition, and discuss any decisions related to their care.
- **Coordinate visits**—If possible, plan family visits to see your loved one in advance. Coordinate schedules to ensure everyone has the opportunity to spend time with them.
- **Support each other**—Encourage open dialog and emotional support. Share your feelings and concerns freely.
- **Respect each other's opinions**—Family members may have different views on the best course of action for your loved one's care. Listen to each other respectfully and try to find common ground.
- **Hold family meetings**—Organize regular family meetings to discuss your loved one's care plan and address any concerns or issues. Avoid I/me/you/your statements and instead use *we/us* language to foster better collaboration.
- **Celebrate milestones**—Find ways to celebrate special occasions and milestones with your loved one. This can help create lasting memories.
- **Seek professional help**—If family conflicts arise or if you need assistance navigating the complexities of long-term care, consider seeking the support of a social worker, counselor, or mediator.
- **Build a network**—You are not alone. There are many champions in your loved one's community. Make friends, compare notes, and ask questions about others who are similarly engaged with their families.

All in a day's work

In managing family relationships, especially when advocating for a loved one in long-term care, embracing flexibility, open communication, and empathy is essential. Challenges and disagreements within the family are inevitable, but how they are addressed can significantly affect the well-being of the loved one and the unity of the family.

Advocates can lead by example, fostering an environment where positive behaviors are encouraged and family members feel heard and respected. Advocates can navigate family dynamics more effectively by understanding different conflict management styles, like those outlined in the Thomas-Kilmann Conflict Mode Instrument, and by prioritizing forgiveness and reconciliation. Balancing the loved one's needs with those of other family members and significant others is vital, ensuring all relationships are nurtured.

While managing family relationships is complex and often challenging, maintaining open lines of communication, respecting different perspectives, and working collaboratively toward the well-being of the loved one can help sustain family harmony and ensure the loved one's needs are met effectively.

Letty Cottin Pogrebin said:

If the family were a boat, it would be a canoe that makes no progress unless everyone paddles.[57]

---

[57] *Top 35 Letty Cottin Pogrebin Quotes (2024 Update) - QuoteFancy.* (n.d.). https://quotefancy.com/letty-cottin-pogrebin-quotes

NOTES

Chapter 14—The Continuing Journey

In this final chapter of *Champions Needed,* we pause and reflect on the crucial role of advocacy in transforming the care landscape for seniors. Throughout our book, we explored the multi-dimensional aspects of advocacy, from understanding the intricacies of the long-term care industry to developing essential communication and problem-solving skills.

Our journey has underscored the significant impact that informed, compassionate, and persistent advocacy can have on the quality of life of our loved ones in care settings. We emphasized the necessity of continuous learning, adaptability, and the power of a positive approach in navigating the complexities of senior care.

We acknowledge the challenges and triumphs encountered by family champions, recognizing that each journey is unique yet universally bonded by a common goal: to ensure dignified, respectful, and personalized care for our elders. As experienced advocates, we've endeavored to provide tools, strategies, and insights to empower families to become effective champions for their loved ones, emphasizing the importance of emotional intelligence, organizational skills, and legal preparedness in this vital role.

By fostering collaborative relationships between families, care providers, and communities, we can build a more compassionate and responsive care system that truly honors each senior's individuality and preferences.

We encourage all champions to carry forward the principles and practices discussed throughout this guide, whether you're one now or will be in the future. The advocacy journey doesn't end here; it's an ongoing commitment to learning, growth, and action.

We urge you to remain vigilant, proactive, and patient in your advocacy efforts, remembering that every small victory contributes to the larger mission of enhancing the care experience for all seniors in assisted living and memory care environments. We must remind ourselves of this every day.

Together, as informed and passionate advocates, we can create meaningful change and ensure that our loved ones receive the respect, care, and joy they deserve in their golden years. Let us move forward with hope, determination, and the knowledge that we're genuinely the champions we aspire to be in the lives of those we hold dear.

NOTES

Last Thought

William Arthur Ward said:

Do more than belong: participate.

Do more than care: help.

Do more than believe: practice.

Do more than be fair: be kind.

Do more than forgive: forget.

Do more than dream: work.[58]

---

[58] "30 Best William Arthur Ward Quotes With Image | Bookey," *Https://Www.Bookey.App/Quote-Author/William-Arthur-Ward,* n.d., https://www.bookey.app/quote-author/william-arthur-ward.

Chapter Summaries

Chapter 1

The chapter emphasizes the importance of advocacy for seniors in long-term care communities, particularly in assisted living and memory care settings. It argues that seniors often need someone to champion their needs as their ability to advocate for themselves diminishes due to age or health conditions. Advocates, whether family, friends, or professionals, are crucial in ensuring that seniors receive proper care, respect, and dignity. The book aims not to criticize the long-term care industry but to encourage individuals to become effective advocates, or 'champions,' for their loved ones. It highlights the necessity of constant communication with care providers and personalized care plans that respect seniors' wishes and individuality. Drawing from their experiences and those of others, the authors intend to provide readers with a clear understanding of the advocate's role, the skills required, and strategies for effective advocacy, aiming to enhance the quality of life for seniors in care communities.

Chapter 2

The chapter focuses on understanding the long-term care industry, highlighting the differences between types of senior living communities and addressing terminology, care models, and industry challenges. The authors advocate for the term "community" over "facility" to emphasize a more inclusive and supportive environment for seniors. They discuss the distinctions between for-profit and non-profit communities, the concept of aging in place, and the continuum of care communities that offer varying levels of service to meet the changing needs of residents. The chapter also describes the specifics of independent living, assisted living, memory care, and skilled nursing care communities, each catering to different resident needs and abilities. Furthermore, it addresses industry-wide challenges such as staffing shortages, increasing senior populations, rising care costs, and varying caregiver training standards. The chapter

 © WatchWorks Management Consulting LLC

emphasizes the importance of being an informed advocate to navigate these complexities and ensure the best care for loved ones.

Chapter 3

The chapter outlines the multifaceted role of an advocate or champion in long-term care, emphasizing flexibility and adaptability as essential traits. The job of an advocate varies significantly based on the changing needs of their loved one, from maintaining routines to managing sudden health crises. The chapter describes an advocate's general responsibilities, which include acting as the primary link between the loved one, their family, and healthcare providers, ensuring the loved one's preferences and needs are addressed, and monitoring the quality of care and living conditions. Skills required for a champion include effective communication, problem-solving, and a strong understanding of medical, legal, and financial aspects related to long-term care. The chapter provides a detailed list of duties and tasks, such as coordinating care, attending meetings, and maintaining records to ensure comprehensive support for the loved one. It also highlights the importance of a positive mindset and continuous learning for successfully navigating the complexities of the advocacy role in long-term care environments.

Chapter 4

The chapter focuses on the importance of emotional intelligence (EQ) for advocates or champions in long-term care settings. It references Daniel Goleman's work to underline the significance of self-regulation, self-awareness, motivation, empathy, and social skills. The chapter suggests that a good advocate must understand and control their impact on others, prioritize others' needs, support motivation, and maintain positivity and authenticity. Emotional intelligence is a lifelong skill crucial in every interaction, particularly in challenging situations within care communities. It provides a framework for applying EQ in practice, including accepting others, asking thoughtful questions, expressing concern, and showing appreciation. The text illustrates the difference between a poor and a better approach when dealing with care staff through a scenario, emphasizing the effectiveness of a calm, understanding, and collaborative approach. It concludes with tips for improving emotional intelligence, such as reading relevant literature, practicing mindfulness, collaborating with care staff, and expanding emotional vocabulary to enhance advocacy and care for loved ones.

Chapter 5

The chapter emphasizes the critical importance of practical communication skills for champions in long-term care settings. It outlines that clear, concise, respectful communication, thoughtful questioning, and active listening form the bedrock of constructive interactions with caregivers and staff. The chapter details strategies to improve communication, such as preparing in advance, maintaining emotional balance, and using the sandwich feedback method for constructive dialogue. It also highlights a scenario contrasting ineffective versus practical communication approaches when addressing care issues, demonstrating how adopting a positive, respectful, and solution-oriented approach can lead to better outcomes for the loved one. The text underlines that every interaction is an opportunity to practice these skills, aiming to foster better care and relationships within the care community.

Chapter 6

The chapter underlines the importance of persistence and tenacity for champions in long-term care settings, drawing inspiration from Benjamin Franklin's adage on the conquering power of energy and persistence. It highlights the necessity of these traits when advocating for a loved one's needs and navigating potential disagreements or misunderstandings within care settings. The chapter emphasizes that understanding and representing the wishes of the loved one are paramount, even when these desires conflict with the advocate's views. It advises on strategies to enhance persistence and tenacity, such as focusing on desired outcomes, managing emotions effectively, and being prepared for multiple interactions to resolve issues. The text illustrates these points with scenarios showing ineffective versus effective approaches, notably in medication management, demonstrating how a well-thought-out, respectful, and collaborative approach can lead to better care outcomes and more robust advocacy for the loved one.

Chapter 7

The chapter focuses on essential problem-solving skills and negotiating for champions in long-term care settings. It emphasizes the importance of adopting diverse strategies beyond one's comfort zone and critical thinking and communication to resolve issues effectively. The chapter suggests problem-solving involves understanding situations from various angles and negotiating solutions that respect all parties' needs. It advises approaching issues by accurately describing problems without bias, identifying root causes, and brainstorming creative solutions. Additionally, it highlights the importance of considering different perspectives and being flexible in negotiations to find mutually beneficial solutions. The text includes scenarios to illustrate effective versus ineffective approaches in addressing care concerns, such as scheduling showers for residents and showcasing how patience, clear communication, and collaboration lead to better outcomes. The chapter encourages champions to maintain persistence, manage emotions, and use clear, concise communication to solve problems and improve the care and quality of life for their loved ones.

Chapter 8

The chapter highlights the essential organization and documentation skills for champions advocating for loved ones in long-term care. It underscores the complexity and significance of managing various documents and information to ensure optimal care and advocacy. Effective organization and meticulous documentation help navigate the administrative and care-related challenges within assisted living and memory care communities. The chapter provides practical tips for improving these skills, including inventorying documents, leveraging technology for storage and access, and creating detailed records of interactions and care plans. It also stresses the importance of being prepared with crucial information, especially in emergencies, as demonstrated in the emergency room registration scenario. Overall, the chapter conveys that thorough organization and diligent documentation are critical for effective advocacy, enabling champions to make informed decisions and communicate effectively on behalf of their loved ones.

Chapter 9

The chapter emphasizes the importance of curiosity and learning agility as essential skills for champions of individuals in long-term care settings. The chapter begins by highlighting the evolutionary and cognitive benefits of curiosity, pointing out how it leads to learning and problem-solving and then relates this to the context of advocacy and caregiving. It suggests that curiosity can be a superpower for champions, driving them to ask open-ended questions that foster understanding and collaboration with care providers. The chapter then transitions to learning agility, described as the ability to quickly understand, adapt to new information, and implement changes. This includes embracing unknown situations, understanding differences, and applying new knowledge to benefit the loved one's care. Strategies to improve curiosity and learning agility involve reading, rehearsal, seeking feedback, reflecting, and experimenting with new approaches. The chapter uses scenarios to illustrate how these skills can lead to more effective interactions and better outcomes in care settings, underlining the necessity of being informed, proactive, and adaptable in advocating for a loved one.

Chapter 10

The chapter underscores the importance of understanding and defending the rights of individuals living in long-term care communities. It draws an analogy to the historical "Don't Tread on Me" motto to emphasize the need for champions to be vigilant and proactive in safeguarding their loved ones' rights. The chapter outlines twenty fundamental rights of residents in such settings, including dignity, respect, privacy, and freedom from abuse and neglect. It highlights the importance of curiosity and learning agility in champions, enabling them to ask critical questions and learn from various situations to better advocate for their loved ones. The text advises maintaining vigilance through regular visits and interactions, employing a curiosity-driven approach to gather information effectively, and addressing issues promptly. It also discusses common areas of complaint within long-term care facilities and guides when and how to file formal complaints with regulatory agencies. The overarching message is that thorough understanding and active defense of a loved one's rights are crucial for ensuring their well-being and dignity in a long-term care setting.

Chapter 11

The chapter addresses the roles and responsibilities of an advocate acting as an agent for a loved one in long-term care, highlighting that this position comes from a legal process that varies by state. The distinction between different types of agents—general, universal, and special—is crucial, each having varying levels of authority. The chapter stresses that while an advocate can also be an agent, there are distinct roles; one may handle financial and legal matters, while another may deal with healthcare decisions. It emphasizes clear communication among family members and other involved parties like healthcare providers and care community staff. Furthermore, the chapter touches on the significance of the power of attorney (POA) and its activation events, including temporary impairment and total incapacitation, underlining the importance of preparatory actions and legal documentation to avoid family disputes and ensure the loved one's wishes are respected, especially in critical end-of-life decisions such as Do Not Resuscitate (DNR) orders.

Chapter 12

The chapter outlines the importance of preparing for individual and community emergencies within long-term care settings. It emphasizes the unexpected nature of health crises and the critical need for champions to be proactive in planning for such events, as residents may face emergencies like falls, sudden illness, or other health issues. The chapter guides maintaining essential documents readily available, understanding community protocols for emergency transport, and discussing preferences regarding emergencies with community management. It highlights community responsibilities to have an emergency preparedness program, urging advocates to review and understand these plans and ensuring they include evacuation procedures and post-emergency processes. The text stresses the significance of advocates being vocal and prepared to safeguard their loved one's rights and well-being during emergencies, illustrating the necessity of being an informed and proactive advocate in unforeseen situations.

Chapter 13

The chapter focuses on understanding and navigating the complexities of family dynamics when advocating for a loved one in long-term care. The chapter emphasizes the importance of attitudes within the family, stating that these deeply ingrained predispositions shape interactions and perceptions among family members. Positive attitudes like empathy, respect, and open-mindedness contribute to healthy communication and understanding, while negative behaviors can create lasting discord. The chapter discusses the necessity for family members, especially advocates, to exhibit flexibility, adaptability, and a collaborative approach to resolve conflicts and ensure the well-being of their loved ones. It stresses that managing family relationships can be one of the most challenging aspects of being a champion for a loved one in care. The chapter also covers conflict management, highlighting the Thomas-Kilmann Conflict Mode Instrument as a tool for understanding and applying different conflict resolution styles. Additionally, it touches on the significance of forgiveness and reconciliation in healing and sustaining family relationships and the balancing act between caring for a loved one and maintaining healthy relationships with significant others. The chapter concludes with practical tips for keeping positive family dynamics, such as regular communication, coordination of visits, and seeking professional help in case of persistent conflicts.

Chapter 14

The chapter serves as a reflective conclusion to the broader discussion on the importance of advocacy in senior care. It emphasizes the transformative impact that informed and compassionate advocacy can have on the lives of seniors in care environments. The authors highlight the essential skills required for

		© WatchWorks Management Consulting LLC

effective advocacy, such as communication, problem-solving, and emotional intelligence, and stress the importance of continuous learning and adaptability. The chapter encourages advocates to persist in ensuring personalized, dignified care for elders and to work collaboratively with care providers and communities. The message is clear: advocacy is an ongoing journey of growth, learning, and action aimed at enhancing the quality of life for seniors in assisted living and memory care settings.

End Notes and Tools

(A) Choosing a Long-Term Care Community

Sponsor	Website
American Association of Retired Persons (AARP)—Assisted Living Checklist—Asking the Right Questions	https://assets.aarp.org/www.aarp.org_/articles/learn/sidebars/3-checklist.htm
National Council on Aging—A Checklist for Moving to Assisted Living	https://www.ncoa.org/advisor/local-care/assisted-living/checklist/
National Institutes on Aging—Long-Term Care Facilities: Assisted Living, Nursing Homes, and Other Residential Care	https://www.nia.nih.gov/health/assisted-living-and-nursing-homes/long-term-care-facilities-assisted-living-nursing-homes
Administration for Community Living—Administration on Aging—Eldercare Locator	https://eldercare.acl.gov/Public/Index.aspx
National Center for Assisted Living—Checklist for Consumers and Prospective Residents	chromeextension://efaidnbmnnnibpcajpcglclefindmkaj/https://www.ahcancal.org/Assisted-Living/Consumer-Resources/Documents/ChecklistforConsumers.pdf

Given the high quality of the available checklists (refer to the websites listed above), we won't *recreate the wheel*. Instead, we'd like to introduce a dozen scenario-based questions you may wish to pose to administrators, staff, and caregivers at prospective LTC communities. They are *what-if* queries the responses to which may be revealing. For simplicity's sake, we're using the name *Sarah* for the loved one.

1) If Sarah can't get to the dining room for any given meal, how will you ensure she gets food?

2) How can Sarah get a drink and snack if she is hungry during the day?

3) If Sarah needs an additional, unscheduled shower, how will you and she handle it?
4) If Sarah needs an additional load of laundry done, how do she and you handle it?
5) What are your target and average response times when Sarah presses her call button?
6) When a community activity starts, how do you remind Sarah and assist her in attending?
7) If Sarah has a handful of visitors simultaneously, what rooms are available?
8) What must be followed if Sarah's visitors wish to dine with Sarah?
9) If Sarah needs a friend or family member to stay overnight, how do she and you handle it?
10) If Sarah appears to have an adverse reaction to a new medication, how do you and she handle it?
11) If Sarah has a minor accident and a small open wound, how do you and she handle it?
12) If Sarah has a medical emergency, what standard process do you follow?

(B) Champion Quick Start Checklist

Becoming a champion for a loved one in assisted living or memory care should be a deliberate decision. With any luck, it won't be thrust upon you suddenly. However, the universe has its operating paradigm, and humans cannot foresee the future well.

As Robert Burns aptly stated, *The best-laid plans of mice and men often go astray.*[59]

We've pondered the challenge of someone being thrust into the role of advocate without much warning or preparation and determined that a few things can be done to get up to speed quickly. We call this our quick start guide.

Before you start down this path, whether your loved one is in an assisted living or memory care community, *please take special care not to overwhelm them with too much information or too many questions at any one time.*

Note: If the loved one is or will be in memory care, these conversations will sound different, perhaps very different from a loved one in assisted living. In our experience, confirming to the cognitively impaired loved one that they're safe, that the community is the right place to be, and that you'll be watching everything closely can go a long way to settling any worry or anxiety.

---

[59] Teahousegarden. "The Best Laid Plans," May 12, 2018. https://www.teahousegarden.com/post/the-best-laid-plans. Note: The original quote from Burn's 1785 poem To A Mouse, is *The best laid schemes o' mice a' men Gang aft a-gley.*

Champion Quick Start Checklist

<table>
<tr><td>

Loved One Meeting
- Express your love, appreciation, and desire to help.
- Review your responsibilities.
- Confirm you have met with other family members.
- Inquire how the loved one is feeling.
- Discuss medications.
- Review the timeline of near-term events.
- Discuss worries or concerns.
- Confirm your next visit or call.

</td></tr>
<tr><td>

Family Meeting
- Confirm you met with the loved one.
- Provide updates on loved one's health and state of mind.
- Review recent/planned changes, esp. new routines.
- Review essential advocate duties and confirm alignment.
- Consider any legal/financial issues.
- Discuss the visit schedule and the family update process.
- Confirm who is accountable in emergencies.
- Summarize key points in an email.

</td></tr>
<tr><td>

Community Administrators Meeting
- Ask questions about the lease, services, and (any) evaluations.
- Confirm your role/duties as the primary advocate.
- Confirm your contact information is on file, with identified back-ups.
- Confirm legal documents are on file, especially POAs and DNR, if any.
- Confirm financial arrangements, including recurring charges and fees.
- Confirm annual statement timing and tax-deductible charges.
- Confirm community policies in emergencies.
- Summarize key points in an email.

</td></tr>
<tr><td>

Community Healthcare Staff Meeting
- Meet with community healthcare providers.
- Confirm your role/duties as the primary advocate.
- Confirm your contact information, with identified back-ups.
- Confirm who is empowered to make healthcare decisions.
- Confirm names and contact information for all providers.
- Confirm medication list, dosages, and timing.
- Confirm daily routines, including meals; review dietary requirements.
- Ask questions about current services, e.g., PT/OT
- Summarize key points in an email.

</td></tr>
<tr><td>

Healthcare and Housekeeping Staff Introductions
- Introduce yourself and confirm your relationship to your loved one.
- Share your phone number and indicate you encourage texts.
- Express your gratitude for taking good care of your loved one.
- Learn the names of healthcare aides.
- Confirm you will (or will not) be a frequent visitor.

</td></tr>
</table>

(C) Champion Readiness Self-Evaluation

This self-evaluation is a simple measure of basic skills, knowledge, and abilities created using the content of *Champions Needed.* It has not been assessed for validity or reliability.

Read the statement in the first column, then score yourself in the second column using the scale below. Scores below the midpoint for the section may indicate areas for development.

1 – Very strongly disagree

2 – Strongly disagree

3 – Disagree

4 – Agree

5 – Strongly agree

6 – Very strongly agree

To what extent do you agree with these statements?

Please use the scoring methodology described on the previous page.

SKILLS	
I am emotionally intelligent.	
I am an effective communicator.	
I am persistent and tenacious.	
I am an effective problem-solver and negotiator.	
I am effective at organizing and documenting.	
I am curious and possess learning agility.	
(Maximum Score = 36 ; Mid-point = 18) SUB-TOTAL	
KNOWLEDGE	
I understand my loved one's medical conditions, treatments, medications, etc.	
I understand health insurance, including Medicare/Medicaid and supplemental plans.	
I understand biological, psychological, cognitive, cultural, and social aspects of aging.	
I understand the laws and regulations governing communities and residents' rights.	
I understand legal terminology and legal matters, e.g., POAs, healthcare directives, etc.	
I understand how to interpret leases, agreements, and other community documents.	
I understand the types of services available in the community.	
(Maximum Score = 42 ; Mid-Point = 21) SUB-TOTAL	
ABILITIES	
I can coordinate medical treatments inside and outside the community.	
I am able to build and maintain solid relationships with community caregivers.	
I can provide insights into my loved one's history, preferences, needs, concerns, etc.	
I can provide emotional support to my loved one, build trust, and respect boundaries.	
I can visit my loved one regularly in person, via phone calls (or other technology).	
I can communicate with family members about my loved one's health and well-being.	
I can shop for my loved one's personal care items, clothing, etc.	
I can ensure my loved one's financial obligations are met on time.	
I can request and attend formal and informal meetings with staff and caregivers.	
(Maximum Score = 54 ; Mid-Point = 27) SUB-TOTAL	
(Maximum Score = 132 ; Mid-Point = 66) GRAND TOTAL	

(D) Training for Caregivers

In *Champions Needed,* we highlighted the necessity for initial and ongoing caregiver training, exacerbated by low unemployment in the U.S. Below are categories and definitions of caregiver training and development priorities.

1) **Alzheimer's and Dementia Support**—Train caregivers in specialized strategies for managing cognitive impairments. Emphasize understanding Alzheimer's and dementia, effective communication methods, behavioral management, and fostering a nurturing environment for residents.

2) **Communication Skills**—Develop caregivers' emotional intelligence and listening skills. Stress the importance of compassionate and respectful interaction with residents, their families, and other service providers.

3) **Emotional and Psychological Wellness**—Equip caregivers to identify signs of emotional distress, depression, and anxiety in residents. Provide tools for engaging residents in activities that enhance their sense of purpose and contribute to a positive living environment.

4) **Incident Management and Escalations**—Educate caregivers on the appropriate steps for escalating resident issues, including when to seek intervention from medical professionals or address non-medical concerns relating to community life.

5) **Legal and Ethical Conduct**—Instruct caregivers on maintaining confidentiality, respecting residents' rights, understanding the boundaries of their roles, and the protocol for reporting abuse or neglect.

6) **Generations**—Offer knowledge of different generations' characteristics, culture, and historical background to foster better understanding and connection between caregivers and residents.

7) **First Aid and Crisis Response**—Provide practical training in first aid for urgent scenarios, including knowledge of DNR (Do Not Resuscitate) orders and handling life-threatening situations like choking or cardiac arrest.

8) **Medication Management**—Ensure caregivers are competent in safely administering medication, understanding common

prescriptions, calculating dosages and storage practices, documenting administration, and recognizing/reporting side effects.

9) **Personal Care**—Cover all aspects of personal resident care, from hygiene and grooming to eating and mobility, including safe lifting and transfer techniques and strategies for preventing falls.

10) **Safety and Emergency Preparedness**—Train caregivers on community-specific safety protocols, including procedures for fire, power outages, and natural disasters, and ensure they know the communication channels and methods for involving family members and emergency services.

(E) Additional Common Scenarios

We don't know of an exhaustive list of scenarios that champions need to be ready to address. However, in addition to the scenarios described within the *Champions Needed* chapters, we have a few more below to consider.

Unexpected charges—Resident lease agreements should specify potential additional service charges when your loved one moves in. For example, salon services are usually not specified but could be billed on the monthly invoice if your loved one asks for that service. The same is true for transportation to/from medical appointments, shopping trips, and delivery of meals when your loved one cannot go to the dining room. Payment for these discretionary services requires minimally a champion's awareness and possibly their intervention.

Suggestions:

- Make a point of asking how services unspecified in the lease will be billed.
- Ask for a list of commonly requested additional services and prices.
- Review each month's invoice to isolate and question new charges.

Annual financial statements and tax preparation—It's customary for long-term care communities to provide annual financial statements to residents and other designated recipients, e.g., champions, accountants, tax preparers, etc. This is also true of insurance companies paying residents or communities under a long-term care insurance contract. Such payments are reported on IRS Form 1099-LTC. While financial statements should be straightforward, most communities must be prompted to provide them.

Suggestions:

- Confer with a tax professional to confirm the information needed for tax filing.
- Discuss the timing for annual statements with the community business manager.

- Store receipts for all unreimbursed medical expenses in a file by category.

Overnight stays—If, as a champion, you do not live near your loved one, it may be necessary (plus convenient and less expensive) for you to stay in the community for one or more nights while visiting. This could be true for other family members as well. Most communities are not overly welcoming of this temporary arrangement and may state as much in a lease agreement. Or the community may limit the number of times this can happen.

Suggestions:

- Ask your questions about an overnight stay as soon as possible.
- Request in writing policy statements that address overnight guests and document same.
- Inform your loved one of what is and what is not possible.

Extended absences—Your loved one may wish to temporarily leave the community for important family or other gatherings, including holidays or vacations. (This is less likely in memory care situations.) Medication management may become a stumbling block for such occasions.

Suggestions:

- Request in writing the process that needs to be followed for a supply of medications.
- Discuss any special considerations with your loved one's physician.
- Review details about the absence of your loved one, especially regarding their safety and comfort.

(F) Medication Management

Seniors living in long-term care facilities can pick any pharmacy they prefer for their medications, but most use the one the community already contracts with. Third-party pharmacies send medicines to the community on a regular schedule. Caregivers authorized to dispense medications to residents use special carts that keep each person's prescriptions separate and safe.

While procedures vary, medicines are usually delivered to communities packed in single-dose blister packs to help dispensers in their daily rounds. Caregivers' teamwork ensures that each resident receives the proper dosages at the correct time. Advocates should be familiar with the dispensers and check in with them regularly.

Advocates must be prepared to facilitate the process when a medication is discontinued, its strength is changed, or a new drug is added. For example, you may need to request that the prescriber fax new prescription information to the community. In some cases, you should hand a hard copy of the new or discontinued medication to staff responsible for administering medications in the community. Follow up the next day to ensure changes have been made.

We're familiar with several companies that perform the third-party pharmacy role. They receive resident prescriptions from medical providers, order refills, and bill insurance. They also package medications by date, day, and time of administration and deliver them to the community. Prescription information is recorded in bespoke software to provide paperless documentation and prevent medication errors.

(G) Long-Term Care Insurance

Long-term care insurance pays for care not covered by regular health insurance, Medicare, or Medicaid. An LTC insurance policy reimburses the cost of care, up to stated maximums, when a covered person requires assistance with Activities of Daily Living (ADLs) due to physical ailments or cognitive impairment. Such policies pay for services in a covered person's home, skilled nursing home, or assisted living/memory care community. Caregivers must meet stated qualifications for expense reimbursement.

There are three common types of long-term care insurance policies:

1. **Individual Policies:** Purchased directly by an individual from an insurer.
2. **Group Policies:** Offered by employers as part of a group plan, often with less stringent underwriting requirements.
3. **Association Policies:** These are provided to members of non-employer associations and are similar to individual policies.

The Federal Long Term Care Insurance Program provides coverage to federal employees, U.S. Postal Service employees, active and retired members of the uniformed services, and qualified relatives. [60]

The younger and healthier you are when searching for suitable LTC coverage, the more likely you are to obtain it and the less expensive it will be. You should take advantage of employer-sponsored plans when available. In 2022, the average annual premium for LTC insurance for a healthy male was $1,200 and $1,960 for a female.

Check out this website for more comprehensive information: https://www.ramseysolutions.com/insurance/long-term-care-insurance-cost.

---

[60] Painter, Kim. "Understanding Long-Term Care Insurance." AARP, February 6, 2024. https://www.aarp.org/caregiving/financial-legal/info-2021/understanding-long-term-care-insurance.html.

Below is a checklist you could use when exploring long-term care insurance:

- **Assess your needs**—Evaluate your potential care needs based on personal and family health history.
- **Understand coverage**—Know what services and facilities are covered under the policy.
- **Benefit amount**—Evaluate the daily or monthly benefit amount against the cost of care in your area.
- **Benefit period**—Decide the length of time you want the policy to pay out benefits.
- **Inflation**—Consider inflation protection to maintain the policy's value over time.
- **Elimination period**—Understand waiting periods before benefits begin and how you'll cover costs.
- **Premium costs**—Review the premium amounts and whether they could change over time.
- **Eligibility requirements**—Know the health conditions for benefits to be paid. Payments are often tied to ADLs or cognitive impairments.
- **Exclusions and limits**—Be aware of what is not covered, such as pre-existing conditions or specific illnesses.
- **Insurer stability**—Check the insurance company's financial ratings and soundness.
- **Shop**—Compare policies from different providers to find the best coverage for your needs.
- **Consult professionals**—Talk to a financial advisor or elder law attorney for tailored guidance.

(H) Resident Rights

Older Americans Act of 1965
https://en.wikipedia.org/wiki/Older_Americans_Act

To meet the diverse needs of the growing numbers of older persons in the United States, President Lyndon Johnson, on July 14, 1965, signed the Older Americans Act (OAA). The OAA set out specific objectives for maintaining the dignity and welfare of older individuals and created the primary vehicle for organizing, coordinating, and providing community-based services and opportunities for older Americans and their families.

Administration on Aging (AoA) https://acl.gov/about-acl/administration-aging

The Administration on Aging (AOA) is the principal agency of the U.S. Department of Health and Human Services designated to carry out the provisions of the Older Americans Act of 1965 (OAA), as amended (42 U.S.C.A. § 3001 et seq.). The OAA promotes the well-being of older individuals by providing services and programs designed to help them live independently in their homes and communities. The Act also empowers the federal government to distribute funds to the states for supportive services for individuals over 60.

Office of Long-term Care Ombudsman Programs
https://acl.gov/programs/Protecting-Rights-and-Preventing-Abuse/Long-term-Care-Ombudsman-Program

The AOA Long Term Care Ombudsman Program began in 1972. Ombudsman programs operate in all states, the District of Columbia, Puerto Rico, and Guam. Each state has an Office of the State Long-Term Care Ombudsman, headed by a full-time state ombudsman. As part of statewide ombudsman programs, thousands of local ombudsman staff and volunteers assist residents and their families by providing a voice for those unable to speak for themselves. For help finding your state's Long-Term Care Ombudsmen program, refer to the National Consumer Voice for Long-Term Care website: https://theconsumervoice.org/get_help.

Office of Elder Justice and Adult Protective Services
https://elderjustice.acl.gov/#gsc.tab=0

The Office of Elder Justice and Adult Protective Services manages the operation, administration, and assessment of the elder abuse prevention, legal assistance development, and pension counseling programs funded through the Older Americans Act and leads the development and implementation of comprehensive Adult Protective Services systems to provide a coordinated and seamless response for helping adult victims of abuse and to prevent misuse before it happens.

Citations and References

"30 Best William Arthur Ward Quotes With Image |
    Bookey," *Https://Www.Bookey.App/Quote-Author/William-Arthur-Ward*,
    n.d., https://www.bookey.app/quote-author/william-arthur-ward.

AARP. "How Continuing Care Retirement Communities Work." AARP, September 5,
    2023. https://www.aarp.org/caregiving/basics/info-2017/continuing-care-
    retirement-communities.html.

AHIP. "Long-Term Care Insurance Covers over 7 Million People Nationwide, New…,"
    November 7, 2023. https://www.ahip.org/news/press-releases/long-term-
    care-insurance-covers-over-7-million-people-nationwide-new-ahip-report-finds.

Alzheimer's Association. "2023 ALZHEIMER'S DISEASE FACTS AND FIGURES SPECIAL
    REPORT THE PATIENT JOURNEY IN AN ERA OF NEW TREATMENTS."
    Https://Www.Alz.Org/Alzheimers-Dementia/Facts-Figures. Alzheimer's
    Association, 2023. https://doi.org/10.1002/alz.13016.

Bandt, Noah. 2022. "Memory Care Reviews, Ratings, and Regulations: How to
    Determine Quality in a Memory Care Facility." March 28, 2022.
    https://www.aplaceformom.com/caregiver-resources/articles/memory-care-
    ratings-reviews-and-violations.

Bar-On, Reuven, and James D. A. Parker. The Handbook of Emotional Intelligence: The
    Theory and Practice of Development, Evaluation, Education, and Application--
    at Home, School, and Workplace. Jossey-Bass, 2000.

Barreira LF, Paiva A, Araújo B, Campos MJ. Challenges to Systems of Long-Term Care:
    Mapping of the Central Concepts from an Umbrella Review. Int J Environ Res
    Public Health. 2023 Jan 17;20(3):1698. Doi: 10.3390/ijerph20031698.
    PMID: 36767064; PMCID: PMC9914432.

Bickerton, James. "Gadsden Flag Meaning Explained and Its Revolutionary Origins."
    Newsweek, August 31, 2023. https://www.newsweek.com/gadsden-flag-
    meaning-explained-1823467.

BrainyQuote. "Benjamin Franklin Quotes," n.d.
    https://www.brainyquote.com/quotes/benjamin_franklin_378118.

Butler, Stuart M. "The Challenging Future of Long-Term Care for Older Adults." JAMA
    Health Forum 3, no. 5 (May 26, 2022): e222133.
    https://doi.org/10.1001/jamahealthforum.2022.2133.

"Caring for Seniors in Long-term Care in an Emergency | HealthLink BC," n.d.
    https://www.healthlinkbc.ca/healthlinkbc-files/caring-seniors-long-term-care-
    emergency.

Carnegie, Dale. How to Win Friends and Influence People. DigiCat, 2022.

CBS News. "A Guide to Long-Term Care Insurance," November 22, 2023.
    https://www.cbsnews.com/news/a-guide-to-long-term-care-insurance/.

"Chapter 28. Spirituality and Community Building | Section 4. Forgiveness and
    Reconciliation | Main Section | Community Toolbox." n.d.
    https://ctb.ku.edu/en/table-of-contents/spirituality-and-community-
    building/forgiveness-and-reconciliation/main.

Cialdini, Robert B., PhD. Influence, New and Expanded: The Psychology of Persuasion. HarperCollins, 2021.

Cobb, Daniel. 2023. "A State-by-State Guide to Assisted Living Regulations." July 18, 2023. https://www.payingforseniorcare.com/state-by-state-guide-to-assisted-living-regulations.

Cohen, Allan R., and David L. Bradford. Influence without Authority. John Wiley & Sons, 2017.

Conlow, Rick, and Rick Conlow. 2022. "50 Persistence Quotes That Inspire & Motivate | Rick Conlow." Rick Conlow. December 11, 2022. https://rickconlow.com/50-persistence-quotes-inspire-motivate/.

"Cost of Long-Term Care by State | Cost of Care Report | Genworth." n.d. https://www.genworth.com/aging-and-you/finances/cost-of-care.html/.

Cottrell, Sarah. "A Year-by-Year Guide to the Different Generations." Parents, January 30, 2024. https://www.parents.com/parenting/better-parenting/style/generation-names-and-years-a-cheat-sheet-for-parents/.

Covey, Stephen R. The 7 Habits of Highly Effective People: Powerful Lessons in Personal Change. Simon and Schuster, 2013.

Denny, Nathan. 2022. "The Biggest Challenges of Long-Term Care in 2023." CareerStaff Unlimited. December 29, 2022. https://www.careerstaff.com/healthcare-staffing-blog/biggest-challenges-of-long-term-care/.

"Dictionary.com | Meanings & Definitions of English Words." In Dictionary.Com, n.d. https://www.dictionary.com/browse/squeaky-wheel-gets-the-grease.

Ebrary. "Challenges for Long-Term Care in the Future," n.d. https://ebrary.net/13565/health/challenges_long-term_care_future.

"Ensuring Quality of Care in Long-Term Care Facilities," December 4, 2023. https://www.ncsl.org/health/ensuring-quality-of-care-in-long-term-care-facilities.

Esposito, Lisa. "Why Ongoing Vigilance Is a Must When a Parent Lives in Memory Care." Https://Health.Usnews.Com/Senior-Care/Articles/. US News and World Report, October 31, 2017. Accessed December 18, 2023. https://health.usnews.com.

EurekAlert! "How Curiosity Changes the Brain to Enhance Learning," October 2, 2014. https://www.eurekalert.org/news-releases/500062.

Geiger, Abigail. "The Whys and Hows of Generations Research | Pew Research Center." Pew Research Center - U.S. Politics & Policy, May 22, 2023. https://www.pewresearch.org/politics/2015/09/03/the-whys-and-hows-of-generations-research/.

Goleman, Daniel. Emotional Intelligence: 25th Anniversary Edition. Bloomsbury Publishing, 2020.

Goyer, Amy. "A Survival Guide to Medication Management." AARP, September 5, 2023. https://www.aarp.org/caregiving/health/info-2020/medication-management.html?cmp=RDRCT-15565558-20201022.

———. "How to Be an Effective Advocate for Aging Parents." AARP, September 5, 2023. https://www.aarp.org/caregiving/basics/info-2020/advocate-for-aging-parents.html.

Gruber, Matthias J., Bernard D. Gelman, and Charan Ranganath. "States of Curiosity Modulate Hippocampus-Dependent Learning via the Dopaminergic Circuit." *Neuron* 84, no. 2 (October 1, 2014): 486–96. https://doi.org/10.1016/j.neuron.2014.08.060.

Hallstrom, Leah. "Total and Percentage of Elderly in Nursing Homes: 2023 Data," December 5, 2023. https://www.aplaceformom.com/senior-living-data/articles/elderly-nursing-home-population#.

Green, H. L. (2020). *POWER OF FORGIVENESS AND RECONCILIATION: Forgiveness is the Sunrise of Reconciliation*. Greenwinefamilybooks.

Injury Facts. "Older Adult Falls - Injury Facts," November 6, 2023. https://injuryfacts.nsc.org/home-and-community/safety-topics/older-adult-falls/#:~:text=Safety%20Topics,-Older%20Adult%20Falls&text=According%20to%20the%20Centers%20for,were%20treated%20in%20emergency%20departments.

Kilmann. "A Brief History of the Thomas-Kilmann Conflict Mode Instrument (TKI)." Kilmann Diagnostics, April 21, 2023. https://kilmanndiagnostics.com/a-brief-history-of-the-thomas-kilmann-conflict-mode-instrument/.

_____. "An Overview of the TKI Assessment Tool." Kilmann Diagnostics, January 8, 2022. https://kilmanndiagnostics.com/brief-overview-of-the-tki-assessment/#:~:text=Kilmann%2C%20co%2Dauthor%20of%20the,underlying%20dimensions%3A%20assertiveness%20and%20cooperativeness.

_____. "Take the Thomas-Kilmann Conflict Mode Instrument (TKI). Take This Assessment Tool and Discover Which of the Five Conflict Modes You Might Be Using Too Much or Too Little... or Just Right." Kilmann Diagnostics, December 24, 2020. https://kilmanndiagnostics.com/overview-thomas-kilmann-conflict-mode-instrument-tki/.

King, S. (2013). *Brag, Worry, Wonder, Bet: A Manager's Guide to Giving Feedback*. iUniverse.

KFF. "Key Issues in Long-Term Services and Supports Quality | KFF," October 28, 2017. https://www.kff.org/medicaid/issue-brief/key-issues-in-long-term-services-and-supports-quality/#:~:text=Recurring%20concerns%20include%20staffing%20levels.

KFF. "The Affordability of Long-Term Care and Support Services: Findings from a KFF Survey | KFF," November 14, 2023. https://www.kff.org/health-costs/poll-finding/the-affordability-of-long-term-care-and-support-services/.

Independence, Forum on Aging Disability, And. "The Challenge." Financing Long-Term Services and Supports for Individuals With Disabilities and Older Adults - NCBI Bookshelf, February 26, 2014. https://www.ncbi.nlm.nih.gov/books/NBK216372/.

Injury Facts. "Older Adult Falls - Injury Facts," November 6, 2023. https://injuryfacts.nsc.org/home-and-community/safety-topics/older-adult-falls/#:~:text=Safety%20Topics,-Older%20Adult%20Falls&text=According%20to%20the%20Centers%20for,were%20treated%20in%20emergency%20departments.

Levins, Hoag. "The Policy and Politics of Long-Term Care: Latest Views on Reform - Penn LDI." Penn LDI, June 28, 2022. https://ldi.upenn.edu/our-work/research-updates/the-policy-and-politics-of-long-term-care-latest-views-on-reform/.

LII / Legal Information Institute. "42 CFR § 483.10 - Resident Rights.," n.d. https://www.law.cornell.edu/cfr/text/42/483.10.

LII / Legal Information Institute. "42 CFR § 483.73 - Emergency Preparedness.," n.d. https://www.law.cornell.edu/cfr/text/42/483.73#:~:text=%C2%A7%20483.7 3%20Emergency%20preparedness.,the%20requirements%20of%20this%20s ection.

Lustbader, Rachel. 2023. "Assisted Living Regulations: A State-by-State Guide." SeniorAdvice.Com. December 21, 2023. https://www.senioradvice.com/articles/assisted-living-regulations-state-by-state.

Mayhew, Jeff. "Roll with the Punches," n.d. https://www.weirdfacts.com/en/origin-of-phrases/origin-of-phrases-r/3963-roll-with-the-punches.

"Memory Care Fact Sheet." n.d. The Joint Commission. https://www.jointcommission.org/resources/news-and-multimedia/fact-sheets/facts-about-memory-care/.

Mohanty, Sarita A. "Millennials Could Soon See Their Parents Become Their Biggest Expense–and American Families Are Woefully Unprepared." *Fortune*, December 30, 2023. https://fortune.com/2023/12/30/millennials-parents-become-biggest-expense-american-families-woefully-unprepared-retirement-personal-finance/.

Molinsky, Andy. "Reinventing the Feedback Sandwich - 5 Different Ways - Andy Molinsky." Andy Molinsky, June 23, 2016. https://www.andymolinsky.com/reinventing-feedback-sandwich-5-different-ways/.

Mollot, Richard J, JD, Sean Whang MPH, Dara Valanejad JD, and The Long-Term Care Community Coalition. Assisted Living: Promising Policies and Practices for Improving Resident Health, Quality of Life, and Safety. eBook. New York, United States of America: The Long-Term Care Community Coalition, 2018. https://nursinghome411.org/ltccc-report-assisted-living-promising-policies-and-practices/.

National Academies Press (US). "Strengthening the Caregiving Work Force." Improving the Quality of Long-Term Care - NCBI Bookshelf, 2001. https://www.ncbi.nlm.nih.gov/books/NBK224489/.

"National Consumer Voice," n.d. https://ltcombudsman.org/issues/residents-rights.

National Institute on Aging. "Specialized Dementia Care in Nursing Homes Linked to Better Outcomes for Residents," September 7, 2023. https://www.nia.nih.gov/news/specialized-dementia-care-nursing-homes-linked-better-outcomes-residents.

Oblates of St. Francis de Sales. "St. Francis de Sales — Oblates of St. Francis de Sales," n.d. https://www.oblates.org/st-francis-wisdom.

O'Connell-Domenech, Alejandra. "The Hill." The Hill, February 7, 2023. https://thehill.com/changing-america/well-being/longevity/3847532-more-people-are-living-to-be-100-heres-why/.

Osmond, C. (2023, June 24). *All Roads Lead to Rome - Origin & Meaning*. GRAMMARIST. https://grammarist.com/proverb/all-roads-lead-to-rome/

Painter, Kim. "Understanding Long-Term Care Insurance." AARP, February 6, 2024.
        https://www.aarp.org/caregiving/financial-legal/info-2021/understanding-
        long-term-care-insurance.html.

Peterson-KFF Health System Tracker. "How Does Medical Inflation Compare to Inflation
        in the Rest of the Economy? - Peterson-KFF Health System Tracker," July 31,
        2023. https://www.healthsystemtracker.org/brief/how-does-medical-
        inflation-compare-to-inflation-in-the-rest-of-the-economy/

Pope, Thaddeus Mason. "Confidentiality and HIPAA." Merck Manuals Consumer
        Version, December 6, 2023.
        https://www.merckmanuals.com/home/fundamentals/legal-and-ethical-
        issues/confidentiality-and-hipaa.

"Protecting, Empowering & Advocating for DC Older Adults," n.d.
        https://www.aarp.org/legal-counsel-for-elderly/.

Quote research. "If Your Only Tool Is a Hammer Then Every Problem Looks like a Nail –
        Quote Investigator®," May 8, 2014.
        https://quoteinvestigator.com/2014/05/08/hammer-nail/.

Rau, Reed Abelson New York Times, Jordan. "Facing Financial Ruin as Costs Soar for
        Elder Care - KFF Health News." KFF Health News, December 4, 2023.
        https://kffhealthnews.org/news/article/dying-broke-facing-financial-ruin-as-
        costs-soar-for-elder-care/.

Rkilmann. "An Overview of the TKI Assessment Tool." Kilmann Diagnostics, January 8,
        2022. https://kilmanndiagnostics.com/brief-overview-of-the-tki-
        assessment/#:~:text=Kilmann%2C%20co%2Dauthor%20of%20the,underlyin
        g%20dimensions%3A%20assertiveness%20and%20cooperativeness.

Rogers, Lisa, and Lisa Rogers. "10 Challenges Facing Assisted Living Facilities."
        Distinctive Living |, May 9, 2022. https://distinctive-liv.com/10-challenges-
        facing-assisted-living-facilities/.

Rowland, Christopher. "Senior Care Is Crushingly Expensive. Boomers Aren't Ready."
        Washington Post, March 24, 2023.
        https://www.washingtonpost.com/business/2023/03/18/senior-care-costs-
        too-high/.

Sammon, Alexander. "The Collapse of Long-Term Care Insurance." The American
        Prospect, October 20, 2020. https://prospect.org/familycare/the-collapse-of-
        long-term-care-insurance/.

Sanghavi, Drishti. "5 LTC Misconceptions That Senior Care Advocacy Is Changing."
        Experience Care: Long-Term Care EHR & Financial Software Solutions (blog),
        September 25, 2023. https://experience.care/blog/5-ltc-misconceptions-
        senior-care-advocacy-is-changing/.

Schier-Akamelu, Rebecca. "What Are the State Requirements for Assisted Living
        Communities? An Overview," January 8, 2024.
        https://www.aplaceformom.com/caregiver-resources/articles/assisted-living-
        violations.

Seo, Krish. "Don't Tread on Me Flag - Origins and Significance." *American Flags* (blog),
        January 23, 2024. https://www.americanflags.com/blog/post/dont-tread-on-
        me-flag-origins-significance.

Smith, Artell. *Engage.Coach.Develop: Building Strong Relationships That Drive
        Individual and Team Performance.* iUniverse, 2023. Page 14.

_____. *No Time to Waste: Microbehaviors: Leveraging the Little Things to Become a Better Leader*. iUniverse, 2023.

"Staffing Challenges in Long Term Care Facilities Continue to Threaten Access to Care for Residents," n.d. https://www.ahcancal.org/News-and-Communications/Press-Releases/Pages/Staffing-Challenges-In-Long-Term-Care-Facilities-Continue-To-Threaten-Access-to-Care-for-Residents.aspx.

"Stephen Hawking Quote: 'Chaos, When Left Alone, Tends to Multiply.,'" n.d. https://quotefancy.com/quote/910026/Stephen-Hawking-Chaos-when-left-alone-tends-to-multiply.

Sy, Payton. "6 Signs It's Time for Memory Care." *US News & World Report*, December 14, 2023. https://health.usnews.com/senior-care/articles/signs-its-time-for-memory-care.

Teahousegarden. "The Best Laid Plans," May 12, 2018. https://www.teahousegarden.com/post/the-best-laid-plans. Note: The original quote from Burn's 1785 poem To A Mouse is *The best laid schemes o' mice an' men/Gang aft a-gley.*

"The CMS National Quality Strategy: A Person-Centered Approach to Improving Quality | CMS," December 13, 2023. https://www.cms.gov/blog/cms-national-quality-strategy-person-centered-approach-improving-quality.

The Editors. "America's Long-Term Care System Is Broken." Scientific American, September 21, 2021. https://www.scientificamerican.com/article/americas-long-term-care-system-is-broken/.

The Joint Commission: https://www.jointcommission.org/resources/news-and-multimedia/fact-sheets/facts-about-memory-care/

Top 35 Letty Cottin Pogrebin Quotes (2024 Update) - QuoteFancy. (n.d.). https://quotefancy.com/letty-cottin-pogrebin-quotes

US Census Bureau, "U.S. Older Population Grew from 2010 to 2020 at Fastest Rate since 1880 to 1890," Census.gov, May 25, 2023, https://www.census.gov/library/stories/2023/05/2020-census-united-states-older-population-grew.html.

W3 Wealth Management. "Long-Term Problems for Long-Term Care Insurance Providers." Business Journal Daily | the Youngstown Publishing Company, June 30, 2022. https://businessjournaldaily.com/long-term-problems-for-long-term-care-insurance-providers/.

"When-and When Not-to Call an Ambulance," n.d. https://www.emergencyphysicians.org/article/er101/when---and-when-not--to-call-an-ambulance.

Wikipedia contributors. "Gerontology." Wikipedia, January 5, 2024. https://en.wikipedia.org/wiki/Gerontology.

Wilson, Keren Brown. "Historical Evolution of Assisted Living in the United States, 1979 to the Present." *The Gerontologist* 47, no. suppl_1 (December 1, 2007): 8–22. https://doi.org/10.1093/geront/47.supplement_1.8.

Additional Resources

Alzheimer's Association
www.alz.org
1-800-272-3900

American Association of Retired Persons (AARP)
www.aarp.org
1-888-687-2277
1-202-434-3524 (Spanish)
1-877-434-7598 (TTY-English)
1-866-238-9488 (TTY-Spanish)

American Healthcare Association and National Center for Assisted Living
www.ahcancal.aspx
1-202-842-4444

American Society on Aging
www.asaging.org
1-800-537-9728

Center for Advocacy for the Rights and Interests of the Elderly (CARIE)
www.carie.org
1-800-356-3606

Justice in Aging
www.justicsinaging.org
1-202-289-6976 (Washington DC)
1-213-639-0930 (Los Angeles CA)

Legal Advocates for Seniors and People with Disabilities (LASPD)
www.mylegaladvocates.org
1-866-785-3328

National Consumer Voice for Quality Long-Term Care
www.theconsumervoice.org
1-202-332-2275 (Washington DC)

National Council on Aging (NCOA)
www.ncoa.org

National Hispanic Council on Aging (NHCOA)
www.nhcoa.org
1-202-347-9733

National Indian Council on Aging, Inc.
www.nicoa.org
1-505-292-2001 (Albuquerque, NM)

Services and Advocacy for LGBT Elders
www.sageusa.com
1-212-741-2247 (New York City, NY)